How To Survive HER MENOPAUSE™

A PRACTICAL GUIDE TO WOMEN'S HEALTH FOR MEN

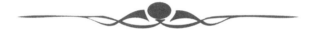

PAT DUCKWORTH

GW00771785

Published by
HWCS Publications
White House, Meeting Lane
Litlington
Royston, Cambs
England SG8 0QF

Bojan Cover design
Pixel Studio

http://pixeldizajn.com/en/

Philip S Marks Editor

Ginger Marks Layout
DocUmeantDesigns

www.DocUmeantDesigns.com

For inquiries about volume orders, please contact the publisher in writing.

Printed in Country
ISBN-13: 978-0-9926620-0-4
ISBN-10: 0-9926620-0-1

DEDICATION

This book is dedicated to the Hot Women who inspired me to write it.

To Linda who suggested it, to Tricia who kept me focused, and to Marina who is a constant inspiration.

CONTENTS

ACKNOWLEDGMENTS

I am grateful to Raymond Aaron for the title of this book.

Thank you to all of the men who told me about their experiences—you know who you are!

Many thanks to my friend Dr. George Grant for his contribution on men's health.

Thanks to the members of Royston Business Network and Melbourn Business Association who were my 'crowd source'.

Many thanks to my editor Philip Marks and formatter Ginger Marks of DocUmeant Publishing & Designs.

As always, many thanks to my husband Alex, for being patient, supportive, and allowing me to bounce ideas off him.

INTRODUCTION

Congratulations! If you are a man reading this book you have either bought it because you are thoughtful and supportive or your partner has bought it for you because she believes that you are thoughtful and supportive. Whichever it is, welcome.

Menopause is a subject that women find it hard to talk about with other women and even harder for them to talk to men about. This is probably because it is associated with ageing and the loss of reproductive function. So it is irrelevant how new or mature your relationship is, what matters is the quality of your communication.

It is not easy to help and support someone who cannot or will not tell you what the problem is. But research has shown that the more supported women going through menopause feel, the better their experience will be. And you don't just get a warm fuzzy feeling from being supportive; being kind and considerate to your partner is also good for your own health.

Menopause is not an illness. It is a natural phase of a woman's life and there are many actions that they can take to ensure that they stay healthy and fit. This is just another phase in our lives and it can be the best phase. Given that we are all living longer, your partner may have over thirty years of post-menopausal life to enjoy with you—so let's get on with it.

But this book is not just for partners of women who are experiencing menopause symptoms naturally. Many women experience these symptoms because of illness or medical interventions such as hysterectomy, radio-therapy, and hormone treatment for cancer. Those circumstances can be particularly challenging for both of you as you deal with the treatment and the side-effects.

You may have heard about Hormone Replacement Therapy (HRT) and assumed that the choice facing your partner is either to take HRT or suffer the symptoms associated with menopause. However the choice is not that simple or that stark and I want to share with you information, advice, and a range of therapy options. The more options your partner has, the less stressed she will be.

Although I have written this book from a woman's perspective, the lifestyle and diet advice and the tech-niques are equally applicable to men. It will also be helpful to you if you are experiencing the symptoms of male menopause, sometimes known as andropause. My friend, Dr George Grant, has written two articles for the chapter on andropause to provide you with more specific advice.

How To Use This Book

It is your choice how you use this book. You can read it all to get a complete picture of menopause or dip in and out of it if you just want to read the bits that relate to something you or your partner is currently experiencing or concerned about.

Chapter 1 is all about effective listening which is essential if you want to support your partner.

Chapters 2 provides you with some definitions and information that will be useful to you and your partner if you want to seek medical advice.

Chapters 3 helps you discover the facts about the male menopause or 'andropause'.

Chapters 4–9 relate to the most common menopausal symptoms. Each chapter includes information, techniques, and comments from real men about their experiences supporting their partners.

In **Chapter 10** I have brought together my Ten Top Tips to control andropause and menopause symptoms.

There are links throughout the book to the bonus journals relating to specific symptoms.

In the resources section I have included some useful book titles and websites if you are interested in further reading on the subject.

CHAPTER 1

WHY WON'T SHE TALK TO ME?

As I have already said, most women do not find it easy to talk about their menopause experience, even to other women. I am guessing that it is not a popular subject for male conversation. A lot of men are squeamish about hearing about women's health issues—especially anything to do with gynaecological matters.

Women often complain that when they try to explain what they are experiencing, men don't listen. In his best-selling book, *Men Are From Mars, Women Are From Venus*, Dr John Gray says that poor communication may arise from the different values that men and women have. Men value 'power, competency, efficiency, and achievement' whereas women value 'love, communication, beauty, and relationships'.

When women talk about their problems they are not necessarily asking for a solution. Part of a woman's strategy for dealing with stress is to share her problems in order to receive support and to nurture her relationships. If your partner talks to you about her menopause symptoms she is not blaming you for them and she does not expect you to cure them. She wants you to listen and understand.

So how do you set up good communication? Here are some skills that you can practice.

1 Rapport skills

Good communication starts with rapport. Rapport occurs when two or more people feel they are in sync or on the same wavelength because they have similar feelings or relate well to each other. Hopefully, there is already a lot of that in your relationship with your partner.

We build rapport with others through our understanding of their world. When we are in rapport with others we unconsciously become more like them and we can do this deliberately if we want to establish and maintain rapport.

You can do this when you are in conversation with your partner by matching her positive body language and breathing pattern. Do not match negative body language because the conversation will go downhill fast! If your partner is sitting down, sit down and turn towards them. If they have their legs crossed, cross your legs. Look at what they are doing with their arms and see if you can do something similar. Notice their breathing pattern and see if you can breathe in and out with them.

It is harder to disagree with someone who is matching you but beware, don't overdo it. You do not want to look like you are patronising the other person.

2 Active listening

You may have heard about 'active listening' as a technique at work. It is about hearing what the other person is really saying. This is much more than just waiting for your turn to speak. It is about giving your full attention to what is being said and confirming that you have understood the content. The three stages of active listening are:

1. Comprehending—this about understanding what the speaker is saying through their verbal and non-verbal communication. This may require confirmation through questioning.
2. Retaining—remembering what the speaker says is essential to your understanding and how successfully you respond. Retention is lost when you make little effort to listen to the speaker's message or engage in some other activity while the speaker is talking.

3. Responding—the speaker looks for both your verbal response and your non-verbal response such as body language.

Becoming an active listener takes concentration, determination, and practice. It takes self-awareness because you need to notice where your thoughts are going and what you are saying with your body language. Being an active listener leads to better communication and better relationships

Here are some top tips for being an active listener for your partner:

- Look at your partner directly.
- Don't be mentally preparing your reply while she is speaking.
- Give your partner your full attention and do not be distracted by environmental factors such as the radio, TV, or mobile phone!
- Watch your partner's body language including gestures, facial expressions, and eye movements.
- Confirm your attention by nodding and making appropriate affirmative sounds such as 'yes', 'ok', or 'uh huh'.
- Check your posture and make sure it is open and inviting.
- Put your own emotions on hold.

- Confirm your understanding by paraphrasing by saying things like 'So what I think you're saying is . . .'
- Ask questions to clarify your understanding such as 'What do you mean when you say you don't feel valued anymore?'
- Do not interrupt your partner to make counter arguments.

Be open and honest in your response.

3 Clean Communication

Clean communication is not about keeping the swearing out of your conversations! It is a technique that was developed in therapy to aid effective communication of issues and to elicit important information. It is a useful tool to use in conversations to enable the speaker to clarify the issues and to help the listener fully understand what is being said.

Many misunderstandings occur because we interpret what is being said from our own experience instead of finding out what the other person is trying to say. For example:

Sue: "I'm finding it difficult to cope with my hot flashes."

Dave: "So, you've got a problem with the sweating?"

Sue: "I didn't think I sweated that much. What are you talking about? Has someone mentioned it to you?"

Dave: "No, I didn't mean that. . . ."

Sue: "Well that's what you said. Now I feel even worse."

Does that sound familiar? A clean language way of approaching that conversation would be to reply using the words that Sue used.

Sue: "I'm finding it difficult to cope with my hot flashes"

Dave: (In a curious, interested tone) "Hmm. Coping with your hot flashes?"

Sue: "Yes. I feel really peculiar when my heart starts to thump."

Dave: "Your heart starts to thump and then what happens?"

Sue: "Well then I start to feel a bit dizzy and then the heat comes up from my chest all the way up to the top of my head."

Dave: "Up to the top of your head?"

Sue: "Yes. It feels good to be able to talk about it. I've been so worried."

This may sound a bit odd or contrived but it is surprising how much more understood the speaker feels and how much more information they give you.

The basic rules are:

- Listen carefully to what your partner says.
- Using a curious tone of voice, repeat back a few words.
- If you need to ask a question do not introduce any of your own words, frame questions around the speaker's words for example: "And then what happens?", "What kind of dizzy is that dizzy?", "Is there anything else about that 'not coping'?"

Using clean communication helps to build rapport, demonstrates that you are listening, and reduces misunderstanding. It will help your partner express what she is feeling and will leave her feeling understood. It's definitely worth giving a try.

A final warning

It would be unfortunate if your partner decided to open up to you on a day when you have had a bad time at work or you are feeling stressed. Stuff happens and those days are not good times to practice your empathy and listening skills.

Unless it is an emergency, if that situation arises it would be better to be straight with your partner. You can say something like "I really want to hear what you have to say but right now it would be difficult for me to listen properly. Let's talk later. How about. . . ."

CHAPTER 2

WHAT IS IT ALL ABOUT?

"My wife had a hysterectomy nearly a year ago. Prior to the operation she was experiencing heavy bleeds because of fibroids. She was finding it exhausting and a bit embarrassing. Because she is still in her 40s, the surgeon put her straight on HRT after the operation and said that he will review the dosage and type in five years.

Obviously, she needed a lot of practical support for about two months after the operation. I work from home so I was able to be there for her. She has recovered now. She has always eaten a healthy diet and exercised regularly so she was in good shape going into the operation and that definitely contributed to her great recovery." Bert

"My wife started taking HRT as soon as she started experiencing menopause symptoms. I thought that was the end of it. Problem solved. Five years later she came off of HRT and immediately started to experience hot flashes and night sweats.

"The HRT was useful because it saw her through a period in her life when she had a high pressure job and needed to be in top form. But I wish I had known that she would still have to go through menopause. I think that should have been made clearer." Colin

You have probably heard menopause referred to as 'the change' or 'time of life'. Menopause is literally the day when a woman has her last menstrual period and that whole phase of a woman's life when she is experiencing a reduction in her reproductive hormones is technically the 'perimenopause'. I have set out the technically correct terms below.

It is generally thought of as a 'women's problem' but men experience some menopausal type symptoms as your hormone levels change in later life. This period is known as 'andropause'. Symptoms can include body shape changes, weight gain, hot flashes, and mood swings. My good friend, Dr George Grant, has written two articles especially for men (see Chapter 3).

Menopause in women can occur naturally as early as forty-five or not until fifty-five but the average age in the UK is fifty-two and fifty-one in the USA. Symptoms can be experienced much earlier as women enter into the perimenopause.

If menopause occurs before the age of forty it is known medically as premature ovarian failure or POF. This occurs in 1 to 4 percent of women. Early menopause can be precipitated by illnesses or medical interventions including hormone treatments, radiotherapy, and hysterectomy, but in 70 percent of cases there is no obvious medical cause.

If your partner's menstrual periods stop before age 40 it is advisable to consult a doctor.

Some Definitions

Various terms are used in connection with menopause and some of them can be a bit confusing. It is important to understand what is generally meant by these terms, particularly if you want to understand your partner or if you need to talk to health professionals.

Climacteric—is not a commonly used term but it refers to the ongoing changes and symptoms that occur during the transition period when ovarian and hormonal production decline. This stage may last fifteen to twenty years between the ages of forty and sixty. It can be compared to the years of puberty and adolescence.

Menopause—is the last menstrual period. Your partner will only know that this was their last period when they have not had a menstrual bleed for at least 12 months.

Perimenopause—is the stage either side of the last menstrual period when women notice most physical changes and when periods may become more irregular.

Post-menopause—relates to the years after the last period up to the end of life. It overlaps with the peri-menopause.

Premature menopause or premature ovarian failure—is menopause that occurs before the age of forty. There may be an identified medical reason or no known reason. If menstrual periods stop before age 40, medical advice should be sought.

Pre-menopause—is the early years of the transition period when menstrual periods may become irregular and sometimes heavier. Other menopause symptoms may be experienced. Generally, this stage starts after the age of forty.

In this book I will mainly be talking about peri-menopause.

Some facts about hormones relating to reproduction

As women approach the end of the reproductive stage of their lives, the supply of eggs decreases and the levels of hormones associated with reproduction begin to decline. This results in the end of menstruation and physical changes to the body.

The hormones involved are:

Oestrogen—*is most commonly thought of as the 'female hormone' although men also produce it. Women produce three forms of oestrogen; oestradiol, oestrone, and oestriol. Oestrogen helps to develop our sexual characteristics and also increases vaginal lubrication and bone formation as well as helping to lift mood.*

Progesterone—*is the key hormone in pregnancy. It helps to maintain pregnancy and prevents further fertilisation. It is the hormone that triggers the menstrual bleed.*

Testosterone—*small amounts of testosterone are produced in the ovaries and adrenal glands. Not much is known about the role of testosterone in women, but scientists believe it helps maintain muscle and bone strength and contributes to sex drive and libido.*

What will her menopause be like?

Every woman's experience of menopause is unique. The easiest way to annoy your partner is to assume that her menopause should be exactly like your mother's/ sister's/friend's. Comments like, *"Do you think you are over-reacting? My mother went through her menopause while looking after my dad and bringing up six children and she never complained,"* will not go unpunished!

There are a number of factors that affect the nature of the menopausal symptoms women experience:

- Genetics. One indication of your partner's possible experience is what happened to their mother and their close female relatives during their menopause. Their experiences can give a clue to the timing and symptoms which might be expected. But remember, your partner only shares 50 percent of her DNA with her mother so her experience may not be the same.
- Diet. The quantity and quality of nutrition will significantly influence the nature of your partner's perimenopause.
- Lifestyle. There are a number of lifestyle factors that have been shown to affect menopausal symptoms including exercise, smoking, and drinking alcohol.

All of this means that women do not have to be victims of their genes. The decisions they make all through their lives about diet, exercise, and lifestyle will have a significant effect on their experience of menopause and their health in later life. It's never too early to plan for a healthy menopause and it is never too late to have a healthy lifestyle.

How will you know if your partner is in the peri-menopause stage?

While many women may have little or no doubt when they start going through the stages of menopause, others may have only minimal discomfort and be unsure about what they are experiencing. This may be a particular issue if the symptoms start to occur before age forty.

The perimenopause symptoms that your partner may experience include:

- Tension
- Mood swings
- Depression
- Forgetfulness
- Poor or interrupted sleep
- Weight change
- Headache
- Tiredness
- Dizziness or faintness
- Heart pounding
- Hot flashes
- Night sweats

- Irregular periods
- Heavier/lighter periods
- Breast tenderness
- Abdominal bloating

If your partner is experiencing regular or intense menopause symptoms, they may want to have a test to confirm the cause. They can purchase a home-test kit to measure their level of Follicle Stimulating Hormone (FSH), the hormone that stimulates your ovaries to produce eggs. A positive test indicates that they may be in a stage of menopause.

Alternatively, advice can be sought from your medical practitioner who may carry out FSH or other tests.

Medically Induced Menopause

Hysterectomy

Hysterectomy is the surgical procedure to remove the womb (uterus). About 60,000 hysterectomies are carried out in the UK every year and over 600,000 in the US.

It is commonly carried out to treat conditions such as:

- Heavy periods
- Long-term pelvic pain
- Fibroids (non-cancerous tumours)
- Cancer of the ovaries, uterus, cervix or the fallopian tubes.

This is a major operation and should only be carried out if other treatments have not been successful. It involves up to five days in hospital and six to eight weeks recovery time.

All hysterectomies involve the removal of the womb but may also involve cervix, ovaries, fallopian tubes, ovaries, lymph glands and fatty tissue.

If the ovaries are left intact there is a chance that the woman will experience menopause within five years of the operation. However if the ovaries are removed as part of the procedure the woman will go into menopause immediately after the operation. This is known as surgical menopause.

Women are usually offered hormone replacement therapy (HRT) after a surgical menopause. This replaces some of the hormones normally produced by the ovaries. HRT is not suitable for everyone and some women experience side effects (see 'HRT or not?')

Despite the statistics quoted above suggesting that this is a commonplace procedure it is, as I have said, major surgery that can impact on the physical, mental and emotional health of the woman. If your partner is offered a hysterectomy there are questions that she will want to ask her doctor such as:

- Do I really need this operation? What are the alternatives?
- How long will the operation take?
- Is there anything I need to do to prepare for it?
- What are the risks?
- Will I have a wound? If so where and how big?
- How long is the recovery period?
- What are the long term effects of the operation?
- Will I have to take any medication after the operation?

If your partner undergoes a hysterectomy be prepared to provide practical and emotional support.

Radiotherapy

Radiotherapy involves the use of high energy X-rays to destroy abnormal tissue, control symptoms, and shrink tumours. It can be applied outside the body using X-rays or within the body through drinking or injecting a liquid containing radioactive material.

Radiotherapy applied to the lower part of the abdomen in premenopausal women usually causes menopause. It can also cause the tissues in the vagina to become stiffer and less stretchy and give rise to vaginal dryness and pain during intercourse.

As with hysterectomy, doctors will usually offer HRT to help overcome the symptoms. They may also suggest lubricants and vaginal dilators.

Hormone Treatment for Cancer

Pre-menopausal women given hormone treatment for breast cancer are likely to experience menopause symptoms.

The treatment plan for breast cancer depends on the stage of the cancer and how far it has spread, the woman's general health and whether she has already gone through menopause.

Some breast cancers are affected by the female hormones, oestrogen and progesterone. Hormone therapy treatment lowers the amount of oestrogen in the body and blocks the action of oestrogen on breast cancer cells.

There are several types of hormonal therapy medicines including:

- aromatase inhibitors, (Arimidex, Aromasin, and Femara)
- selective oestrogen receptor modulators, (Tamoxifen, Evista, and Fareston)

- oestrogen receptor downregulators (Faslodex)

The dose and the period of time that it will need to be taken depends on the individual and their response to the medication. Recent research has concluded that some women need to take Tamoxifen for up to ten years.

If your partner is experiencing side effects from hormone treatment she should discuss it with her doctor, cancer specialist, or breast care nurse.

HRT or not?

You may be thinking 'What is the problem with menopause? Surely she could just take HRT.' Time to learn a bit more about the pros and cons of HRT.

Hormone Replacement Therapy (HRT), also referred to as Hormone Therapy, has been available since the 1930s. The earliest prescription drug for oestrogen was called Premarin which was an oral medication made from the urine of pregnant horses. This was followed by a synthetic form of progesterone called Prempro. Newer medications combine oestrogen and progestin.

Initially it was thought to be safe for women to start taking HRT at the onset of menopausal symptoms and to stay on it for the rest of their lives. Following the report of the Women's Health Initiative in 2002 it was recommended that women only stay on HRT for the short term (e.g., 5 years) due to the potential health risks such as increased risk of heart attacks and breast cancer. As soon as you stop taking HRT you may experience menopause symptoms no matter what age you are.

Most women seek HRT to control hot flashes and night sweats but some also consider it because they think that it will keep their hair and skin looking good and also give them more energy and a better sex drive. Research published in 2003 (NEJM, 2003) concluded that "In this trial in postmenopausal women, oestrogen plus progestin did not have a clinically meaningful effect on health-related quality of life."

There is a large range of HRT products available which are manufactured from a variety of ingredients. They can be administered in a variety of forms:

- Implants. A pellet containing a six month supply of oestrogen is inserted under the skin of the lower abdomen.
- Tablets. This is the most common way of taking HRT where oestrogen is taken every day and progestogen is taken from day 15 to day 25 of the cycle.
- Skin patches. Skin patches deliver hormones directly to the bloodstream through the skin and, as with the implants, this means that the required dose is lower, reducing side effects.
- Vaginal rings, pessaries, and creams. Preparations containing oestrogen to be applied di-

rectly to the vagina can be prescribed to ease symptoms such as vaginal dryness, itching, burning, or discharge.

- Gels and creams. Oestrogen gels and creams rubbed on to the skin are absorbed easily and enter into the circulatory system.

HRT can have unpleasant side effects including depression, skin rashes, hair loss, vomiting, bloating, and a cystitis-like syndrome. It is unsuitable for some women, particularly those who smoke, have high blood pressure, benign breast disease, endometriosis, pancreatitis, epilepsy, or migraines.

Bio-Identical Hormone Therapy (BIHT)

Bio-identical hormones have been prescribed in the US for many years but have only recently become available in the UK. They have structures identical to human hormones and are mostly derived from plant sources including soy or Mexican yam root. Although they are considered to be 'more natural' than other HT products, the plant compounds undergo synthetic processing to obtain the hormones used.

As with HT, BIHT can take a variety of forms including tablets and creams to suit different symptoms. Practitioners will normally aim to treat with the lowest dose for the shortest period of time.

It is possible to purchase bio-identical hormones over the internet but it is inadvisable to self-medicate. These are drugs—they carry risks and the chance of side effects. Always discuss the options with your doctor.

Self-Advocacy

If your partner is experiencing moderate or severe menopausal symptoms she may be considering some form of hormone therapy. It is debatable whether BIHT is any more natural or lower risk than HRT. All forms of HRT have a long list of contraindications and possible side effects.

The important thing in making this decision is to be well informed about the benefits and the risks before discussing the options with a medical practitioner. Good communication between the doctor and the patient is a key to effective treatment.

There are some references for further reading in the Resources section at the end of this book.

CHAPTER 3

DO MEN HAVE A MENOPAUSE?

"I am in my late 50s and I have started to experience problems getting and keeping an erection. I would like some advice but it's not a problem that I feel I can talk to other men about and I don't want to go to the doctor.

"I think part of the problem may be the relationship that I am in. We have had a lot of pressures recently and we aren't communicating well. Apart from that I am generally fit and healthy. I eat a good diet and take regular exercise." Raj

"Hot flushes. I never called them that. But then I never really knew what was happening. A few times a week, or once every few weeks, I would

break out in a sweat. Sometimes in the day, sometimes at night. I felt hot, but not uncomfortable, and it would pass in an hour or so. It didn't stop me doing anything, but I am sure it looked odd to people if my shirt was wet with sweat patches on a cold day.

"There didn't seem to be any trigger or cycle that I could find. It lasted about three years and then tailed off. It was only when a friend said he had had a similar experience that I belatedly added 2 + 2 to conclude it was andropause." Matthew

Andropause is often referred to as the male equivalent of the menopause. Before you dismiss the idea of the male menopause, think about the hormonal changes you have had in your life. There was the physical and emotional turmoil of puberty when your hormones made huge changes to your body—and your feelings for the girl next door.

Since those teenage years the balance of your hormones has changed and levels of the sex/reproduction hormones have gradually diminished. Research has shown that hormonal imbalance affects 20 percent of men over the age of 50. So what is going on?

As you move into your late forties and fifties, it is natural for the levels of your reproductive hormones to start to decline. Most significant is the reduction in the level of testosterone. Testosterone is a hormone that is produced in the testes. It builds you up and is essential to men's health.

However, unlike menopause for women, testosterone deficiency syndrome (TDS) does not affect all men. Where it does, TDS can give rise to symptoms such as:

- General fatigue
- Changes to body shape
- Erectile dysfunction
- Loss of interest in sex
- Loss of bone density
- Hot flashes/night sweats
- Palpitations
- Hair loss
- Low mood/depression

There are some factors that increase the risk of TDS for example, trauma to the testes and diabetes. Living an unhealthy lifestyle with poor diet, little exercise, alcohol abuse, and stress will also increase your chance of this condition.

There are tests and treatments available for TDS and if you are experiencing frequent or intense symptoms you should consult your medical practitioner. There is an Andropause Symptoms Record in the Resources section of this book. I have also included the details of useful websites on the subject.

If you are experiencing some of the symptoms listed above, the nutrition and lifestyle advice contained in this book would be helpful to you as well as your partner.

Natural Solution for Enlarged Prostate by Dr George Grant

Most men between the ages of 40 and 45 experience a gradual increase in prostate size. An increased urge to urinate and weak urinary flow are effects of prostatic hyperplasia and are common signs of an alteration in the male hormonal balance.

Close to 50 percent of men in their fifties and as many as 75 percent of men between the ages of sixty and seventy suffer from benign prostatic hyperplasia (BPH).

BPH causes a narrowing of the urethra and promotes bladder problems. The exact cause of prostate enlargement is not fully understood. Although the body normally turns ordinary testosterone into a very potent form called dihydrotestosterone (DHT), it can cause an enlargement when there is too much DHT. Wrapping around the urethra, the tube that allows urine to exit the bladder, a swollen prostate gland acts like a clamp, sometimes resulting in problems with urination.

Symptoms of BPH include:

- Getting up frequently at night to urinate.
- More frequent urges to urinate.
- Diminished, weakened stream.
- Feeling of incomplete emptying of the bladder.
- Pain and burning sensation.

Left untreated, prostate problems can prevent the bladder from emptying itself completely. As the volume of residual urine increases, a humid environment creates the perfect conditions for the proliferation of bacteria. This can cause urinary tract infections, with symptoms of pain and fever. The final stage of benign prostatic hyperplasia can cause acute urine retention which is extremely painful.

Natural Solutions to BPH:

Saw palmetto, a very beneficial and well-studied herb, provides great therapy for the enlarged prostate. In fact, one study showed significant improvement in 45 days with only mild or no side effects.

Hydrangea root or horsetail are often used to reduce the inflammation of the prostate gland. Nettle root tincture or capsules are also helpful. In fact, scientific studies have proved its ability to diminish this enlarged gland. Amounts used in successful studies range from 6-12 mL of tincture per day in divided doses, or 120 mg capsules twice a day.

The mineral zinc may halt the processing of testosterone into DHT and thus may prevent or even reverse the condition. Pumpkin seeds from your garden are an excellent source of zinc, especially if you fertilize with kelp, and may contain other helpful substances as well. Eating 2 ounces of pumpkin seeds per day significantly boosts your zinc intake. Some people prefer to take zinc supplements for BPH. If you decide to supplement with zinc, use no more than 50 mg per day for three months and include a copper supplement of 2 mg per day. These two minerals compete for absorption zinc will win out and cause a copper deficiency if you're not careful. Look for a zinc supplement that includes copper.

Keep in shape and maintain an active lifestyle by walking or doing some exercise to slow down the aging process, one of the main causes of BPH. Research suggests that pygeum (P. africanum) helps to reduce nocturnal symptoms, hesitancy, and urgency (30-40 percent reduction in symptoms). Lycopene, vitamin D, pomegranate juice, and omega-3 fatty acids are supplements that have been shown to have a protective role in the prevention of prostate cancer.

Top Tips:

- Avoid bicycling, the sitting position compresses the prostate.

- Cold temperatures exacerbate the symptoms. Make sure you keep the abdomen warm.

- Do not drink too much before going to bed to prevent night time visits to the bathroom.

- Don't ignore the need to go to the bathroom. Fully empty the bladder. Void your bladder every time you urinate.

- Constipation can aggravate the prostate problems, so it is important to have good bowel health.

- Stop smoking.

- Pay attention to certain prescription drugs—diuretics, antispasmodics, tranquilizers, and some anti-depressants worsen BPH.

- After age 45, do not neglect yearly medical exams.

- Food

  o Avoid drinking chilled beverages or iced cocktails. Cold drinks do more harm than good and can cause a sudden blockage of the urinary track, resulting in difficult and painful urination.

  o Reduce alcohol intake.

  o Reduce caffeine intake; coffee substitute is a great alternative.

  o Drink plenty of water and lemon. Empty bladder regularly.

  o Avoid substances that irritate the prostate gland—pepper, hot peppers, and spices

  o Maintain a diet high in fibre, vitamins, and minerals.

o Avoid or reduce saturated fats such as those in most processed foods, dairy products, red meats, and hard fats. Replace by cold pressed vegetable oils.

o A diet low in both fat and red meat and high in protein and vegetables, as well as moderate alcohol consumption, may reduce the risk of symptomatic BPH.

o Vegetarian foods, raw fruit and vegetables, soy products, and pulses including linseed are useful in bringing relief.

2 Erectile Dysfunction by Dr George Grant

Erection problems are not always related to erectile dysfunction per se. Other factors related to physical and emotional health can lead to temporary issues in the bedroom, including:

1. Alcohol use: While a drink or two can help to break the ice and move things toward the bedroom more quickly, overdoing it can have an unintended and unfortunate effect. Alcohol is a depressant, or downer, and one of the victims of the downer effect is the ability to become erect. Men who have romantic intentions for the evening should keep their consumption to no more than two drinks in order to avoid an embarrassing end to an evening.

2. Smoking: Smoking wreaks havoc on the body in numerous ways, including hardening and narrowing the blood vessels, interfering with neural activity and reducing stamina. Crushing out the butts is a proactive step toward overall better health, not to mention improved sexual ability.

3. Stress: The pressures of maintaining a job, caring for a family, studying for exams, or anything else that keeps a man up at night can cause chemical stress reactions that tend to interfere with erectile ability. Reducing stress or finding better ways to cope can help to improve his ability to react to stimulation.

4. Poor circulation: Reduced circulation to the penis, whether due to excess body fat, reduced heart function, or just sitting at a desk for too long can restrict blood flow and result in at least temporary reduction in erectile action.

5. Depression: Depression and other emotional or mood disorders can manifest as loss of erectile ability; on the flip side, loss of erectile function can actually lead to depression. In either case, treating the depression with counselling and or medication may help.

6. Relationship issues: Whether faced with partner conflict or just an old relationship in which the sex just does not feel new and exciting any more, a man who is not feeling comfortable with his mate may not feel aroused every time the occasion calls for it. Couples counselling—or even a change in partners—might provide the answer in this case.

7. Medications: Certain prescription medications can lead to loss of function. When medications are in the mix, talking to a doctor about an alternative may help to resolve the issue.

8. Peyronies disease: This disease causes fibers and plaques to appear in the genitals, interrupting blood flow.

9. Cancer: Cancer can interfere with nerves or arteries that are vital to erection.

10. Surgery: Surgery to the pelvis, and especially prostate surgery for prostate cancer, can damage the nerves and arteries that are required to gain and maintain an erection.

11. Spinal cord or pelvic injury: The nerves that stimulate erection can be cut by injury.

12. Hormonal disorders: A lack of testosterone (male hormone or androgen) can result from thyroid disorders.

13. Performance anxiety: Most men have had erection problems at some point due to worrying about performing well during sexual intercourse. If this happens often, the anticipation of sex can trigger nervous reactions that prevent erection, setting up a vicious cycle.

14. Situational psychological problems: Some men have problems only in certain situations or with certain people. In troubled relationships, men may be unable to achieve erection with their partner but have no problem away from home.

15. Sexual aversion: Being repelled by sex is rare. It is most common in people who suffered child abuse and those who have been brought up in strict religious surroundings. Aversion can also exist in homosexuals or bisexuals who attempt to lead a heterosexual life against their basic inclinations.

16. Illnesses: These can include heart disease, clogged blood vessels (atherosclerosis), high LDL cholesterol, high blood pressure, diabetes, obesity, metabolic syndrome (a condition involving increased blood pressure, high insulin levels, body fat around the waist), Parkinson disease, multiple sclerosis, low testosterone.

17. Drugs: The following can cause erectile dysfunction: alcohol, antianxiety medications, anti-cancer medications, cocaine, estrogens, ganglionic and adrenergic (beta) blockers, MAOI and tricyclic anti-depressants, narcotic pain relievers, narcotics, thiazide diuretics that are prescribed to control high blood pressure (and other blood pressure medications, such as calcium channel blockers) and sedatives.

Treatment

Currently, virtually any man who wishes to have an erection can obtain it, regardless of the underlying cause of his problem. Many reasonable treatment options exist. Your first step is to find a well-trained, experienced, and compassionate doctor who is willing to take the time to understand you as well as to fully examine you to discover the cause of erectile dysfunction. Together, you and your doctor can then discuss possible treatments.

Allopathic Treatment:

1. Cialis, Levitra, Staxyn, Stendra, and Viagra work by a similar mechanism to cause erections. There are subtle differences in how long the drug works and how quickly it works.

2. Testosterone, bromocriptine, and cabergoline are hormonal treatments that may help with erectile dysfunction. Inadequate production of testosterone is not a common cause of erectile dysfunction; however, when ED does occur due to decreased testosterone production, testosterone replacement therapy may improve the problem.

Natural Treatment:

1. Horny goat weed is an herb that has been a traditional remedy in China for centuries. It is used for low libido, erectile dysfunction, fatigue, pain, and other conditions.

2. Arginine. The amino acid L-arginine, which occurs naturally in food, boosts the body production of nitric oxide, a compound that facilitates erections by dilating blood vessels in the penis.

3. DHEA, a hormone that the body converts to testosterone and estrogen, can help alleviate some cases of ED.

4. Korean red ginseng has long been used to stimulate male sexual function, but few studies have tried systematically to confirm its benefits.

5. Ginkgo biloba. Known primarily as a treatment for cognitive decline, ginkgo has also been used to treat erectile dysfunction, especially in cases caused by the use of certain medications.

6. Propionyl-L-carnitine and acetyl-L-carnitine were found to enhance the effectiveness of sildenafil, and result in improved erectile function, sexual intercourse satisfaction, orgasm, and general sexual well-being compared to Viagra alone.

6. Zinc. Significant depletion of the mineral zinc, associated with long-term use of diuretics, diabetes, digestive disorders, and certain kidney and liver diseases, has been shown to lead to erectile dysfunction.

7. Ashwagandha. The herb ashwagandha (Withania somnifera) is sometimes called Indian Ginseng because it is thought to have similar effects on the body. It is thought to increase energy, stamina, and sexual function. No studies, however, have examined whether it is effective for erectile dysfunction in humans.

8. Yohimbe The bark of the West African yohimbe tree is a source of yohimbine, a compound that has been

found to stimulate blood flow to the penis, increase libido, and decrease the period between ejaculations.

9. Damiana is a plant native to Mexico and the southern United States. It has been widely used as an aphrodisiac in Mexico for men and women.

10. Tribulus terrestris is an herb that has been used in the traditional medicine of China and India for centuries. It was only in the mid–90s when Eastern European Olympic athletes claimed that tribulus contributed to their success that tribulus became known in the North America.

11. Muira puama, also called potency wood is a small Brazilian tree that grows across the Amazon river basin. It has a long history of use in Brazilian folk medicine as an aphrodisiac.

12. Tongkat Ali is a tree native to Malaysia, Thailand, and Indonesia. It was dubbed the Asian Viagra

13. Maca is often touted as an aphrodisiac and a natural means of improving sexual performance and fertility. Although few scientific studies have tested Maca medicinal effects, some research suggests that maca may offer certain health benefits.

Dr. George Grant, Ph.D., IMD *The Caring Doctor* Specialist in Integrative Medicine, Nutrition, Biofeedback, Pain & Stress www.academyofwellness.com; www.your101ways.com

CHAPTER 4

WHY IS MY WOMAN SO HOT?

"My partner has been experiencing frequent and severe hot flashes and night sweats for several years. I notice it during the day because we work together. She often uses a fan and wears layers of clothes to take-off and put back on depending on her temperature. But it has more impact for both of us at night. The duvet is thrown on and off. I feel really sorry for her but it does also disturb my sleep. We both run our own businesses and need a proper night's sleep.

"She has been much better since she started using cool visualisation recordings and other techniques that [Pat Duckworth] has taught her. It would probably help if we cut down on the wine!" Jo

If you are sleeping next to a woman who experiences hot flashes you know just how hot and uncomfortable it can be. Hot flashes are one of the most common symptoms that send women to see their doctors when they are going through the perimenopause.

About 60 percent of women experience hot flashes and/or night sweats and of those, 70 percent experience them for a year and 30 percent for about 5 years (Foxcroft, 2009) So it is surprising that so little is known about what causes them and what is going on inside the body when a woman has one.

During a hot flash the blood vessels dilate, increasing the flow of blood to the skin, most noticeably to the face, neck, and chest, but also in the back. A rise in temperature is accompanied by sensations of heat, sometimes overwhelming, followed by sweating and cooling down. Some women also experience increased heart rate, dizziness, faintness, and nausea. A hot flash generally lasts between 3 and 5 minutes.

The implications of hot flashes have been subject to many research projects but the results are not consistent. One study has shown that women who suffer from hot flashes and night sweats may be at lower risk for cardiovascular disease and stroke. "While they are certainly bothersome, hot flashes may not be all bad," according to Northwestern Medicine endocrinologist Emily Szmuilowicz, MD, who is lead author of the study, "Our research found that despite previous reports suggesting that menopause symptoms were associated with increased levels of risk markers for heart disease, such as blood pressure and cholesterol, the actual outcomes tell a different story."

Other studies suggest that the parasympathetic nervous system works less well during hot flashes (Goodwin, J. 2012). Although this effect is transient, as the parasympathetic nervous system regulates the body at rest, more research is being done in this area.

The intensity and duration of hot flashes varies from woman to woman. At their mildest, a hot flash can be something that a woman is aware of without any particular discomfort or embarrassment. At their most severe a hot flash can give rise to copious sweating and a sensation like the onset of a heart attack.

Not every woman who has hot flashes also has night sweats but if they have hot flashes at night they can wake up hot and drenched in sweat. Night sweats may occur several times a night and can result in interrupted sleep. It is important to note that night sweats can be related to non-menopausal issues such as stress and your partner should consult a doctor if she is unsure of the cause.

Several recent studies have concluded that women who lose weight could experience fewer menopausal symptoms including hot flashes. A study by the journal, *Menopause*, found that women who followed a low-fat, high fruit, vegetable and fibre diet lost weight and had significantly reduced hot flashes and night sweats. One reason for this could be that body fat can prevent heat loss because it acts as insulation.

Sleep

As already mentioned, hot flashes and night sweats can lead to poor or disrupted sleep both for your partner and you. It's not easy to sleep when you are lying next to someone who is thrashing about and is as hot as a furnace. Many women report disrupted sleep and tiredness as their biggest menopause problem.

Good sleep is essential to good physical, emotional, and mental health for men and women. During a good night's sleep you have balanced periods of slow-wave sleep, where your body carries out physical housekeeping, and rapid eye movement sleep (REM) where your brain sorts out memories from the day.

Poor sleep is characterised by longer periods of REM and shorter slow-wave sleep. This type of pattern can lead to you feeling tired when you wake up in the morning because your body has not had sufficient rest.

Good sleep is important because it:

- Rejuvenates the body
- Enhances health:
    - Lowers risk of heart problems
    - May prevent cancer
    - Reduces stress
    - Reduces inflammation
    - May help to control weight
- Aids memory
- Energises
- Lifts mood

People vary in how much sleep they need. Some people believe that they are sleep deprived if they are not getting eight hours sleep a night or as much sleep as they used to when they were younger. However, not everyone needs eight hours sleep—Margaret Thatcher famously was said to need only four hours. Most people find that as they age they need less sleep.

It is easy to worry too much about whether you are getting enough sleep. If you function pretty well during the day, you're doing fine and you can stop lying in bed worrying about not getting enough sleep.

What you can do to improve sleep

The good news is that over time, hot flashes get milder and less frequent and, for most women, they eventually disappear altogether. If they are particularly severe and debilitating your partner may want to consider medical treatment such as HRT or selective serotonin reuptake inhibitors (SSRIs). Some medical practitioners prescribe antidepressants for hot flashes. If your partner's doctor suggests this encourage her to ask about the benefits, risks, and side-effects.

Otherwise there are some diet and lifestyle changes that may help. Before you or your partner start to make any changes, it is helpful to identify any patterns of good or poor sleep by keeping a sleep journal for a week.

You can download a 'Sleep Journal' template at www.hotwomencoolsolutions.com.

Diet

There are changes that your partner can make to her diet that will help to balance her hormones. These would also be healthy for you so there is no need to have separate meals.

- Eliminate dietary triggers—Common triggers include sugar, caffeine, chocolate, alcohol, and spicy foods.

- Drink more water or cool non-carbonated drinks.
- Include phytoestrogens in the diet for example:
    o Isoflavines—soya, chickpeas, lentils, and kidney beans
    o Lignans—flaxseeds (linseeds), sesame seeds, sunflower seeds, brown rice, oats, broccoli, and carrots
    o Coumestans—found in sprouted mung beans and alfalfa beans
- Eat more omega-3 fatty acids—found in sardines, salmon, mackerel, and flaxseeds (linseeds).

For best effect eat organic, unprocessed foods whenever possible.

Including foods that contain the hormone tryptophan in your diet can help to encourage good sleep. These foods include turkey, chicken breast, cheese, soy beans, and tuna. They are most effective when eaten with carbohydrate. So a good bedtime snack is cereal with milk, peanut butter on toast, or cheese and crackers.

Drinking alcohol before bedtime is best avoided as it can trigger night sweats. An alcoholic drink before bedtime may relax you but it can cause disrupted or disturbed sleep. It also keeps you from entering the deeper stages of sleep which can lead to waking up feeling tired.

Sleep medication

In the UK, more than 10 million prescriptions are given for sleeping pills every year. Medication offers only short term relief because sleeping tablets treat the symptoms of poor sleep and not the causes. Medical practitioners are advised to prescribe drugs only after considering non-drug therapies

If you or your partner are thinking of taking sleeping tablets or are already taking them, there are some things you might want to consider. Not all sleeping pills are the same. Each class of sleep aid works a bit differently from the others, and side effects vary.

It's important to ask key questions before choosing your sleep medicine.

o   *How long does it take for the sleeping pill to take effect?*
o   *How long do the effects last?*
o   *What's the risk of becoming dependent on the sleeping pill, physically or psychologically?*

Non-prescription medicines

There are many over the counter remedies available at a pharmacy. The common ingre-

dient in all these pills is an antihistamine, which causes drowsiness. So whatever you choose you are essentially getting the same type of medicine.

Always check with your doctor before taking over-the-counter medication. Even commonly available sleeping pills can cause side effects and interact with other medication you are taking. So exercise caution and take only as directed by your doctor.

Complementary therapies

There is a range of complementary therapies that can help alleviate sleep problems for you or your partner.

Aromatherapy A few drop of some essential oils added to a warm bath before bed can help to ease sleep problems. Lavender oil is anti-inflammatory and has a mildly sedative effect. Chamomile and ylang-ylang also appear to improve sleep. nb Some people may experience irritation when using essential oils. Essential oils should never be applied directly to the skin.

Herbal Remedies There is some evidence that the herb valerian is effective for insomnia. Passionflower, hops, lavender, lemon balm, and Jamaica dogwood are also traditionally used to help you sleep, but their benefits have not been proven in medical trials. If you are taking any other medication, check with your medical practitioner or pharmacist before taking any herbal remedies.

Homeopathic remedies Homeopaths do not usually prescribe remedies for individual symptoms, instead the remedy is to treat the whole person. Some common remedies for sleep disorders include:

- Arnica—for overwork and when the bed feels hard and uncomfortable
- Aconite—for acute insomnia caused by shock, fright, bad news, or grief
- Kali phos—night terrors or exhaustion from stress or overwork
- Lachesis—night sweats
- Pulsatilla—early waking with over-active mind
- Sepia—difficulty falling asleep, night sweats

Bedroom changes

If you are experiencing poor or interrupted sleep, check the quality of your bedroom environment. Your bedroom should be a sleep haven. Remove the TV, computers, smart phones, etc from the bedroom so that there are no distractions from sleep.

Keep your bedroom cool and well ventilated. Most people sleep best in a room that is dark and quiet. Also, consider whether you need a more comfortable mattress or different pillows. Sleep under a light duvet or loosely woven blanket. You could consider having separate single duvets or covers so that you can both have the correct temperature.

Self-hypnosis

Self-hypnosis is a useful technique for getting back to sleep during the night.

1. Settle down and make any adjustments to be completely comfortable.
2. Close your eyes and focus on your breathing without trying to change it. Notice your thoughts and let them just slip away.
3. Send your attention around your body noticing any sensations or aches and pains without judging them or putting any meaning to them.
4. Start letting go of any tension in your body. Beginning at your toes, tense them and then relax them. Flex your feet and relax them. Move up your body tensing and relaxing your muscles.
5. When your attention gets to your head, clench and relax your jaw. Imagine your cheeks and then the top of your head being gently massaged.
6. Continue to breathe slowly and deeply. Recognise how relaxed you are feeling. You may feel like you are floating or sinking. You can use that feeling and send yourself a positive message by repeating an affirmation to yourself for example 'I am cool and comfortable.' or 'I am drifting off into deep and refreshing sleep.' or 'I am

successful and positive.' Repeat your statement as many times as seems appropriate.

7. If you are going through this process at night, you can let yourself drift off to sleep. If you are relaxing during the day you can let your consciousness return to the room, noticing your surroundings and saying out loud 'Wide Awake' or 'Back in the room.'

If you find this technique difficult, you could buy a pre-recorded hypnosis CD. If you can, listen to a sample before you buy so that you know whether the voice in the recording is right for you. Some voices are like finger nails on a blackboard!

Your Bonus

You can download a relaxation/hypnotic recording to aid better sleep at www.hotwomencoolsolutions.com.

CHAPTER 5

SHOULD I BE WORRYING ABOUT HER WEIGHT?

Body Changes

You may have noticed your partner's body shape changing. Your own body shape may be changing too as you mature.

Just as during puberty, hormonal changes during perimenopause bring about changes to a woman's weight and body shape. Men also experience changes to their body shape as they get older. At this stage of life, the metabolic rate of both you and your partner will be slowing down and you may be naturally losing muscle which helps you burn off fat.

During this phase of a woman's life her ovaries produce less oestrogen and her body tries to compensate by manufacturing oestrogen elsewhere to protect the body against osteoporosis. The fat around the middle of the body is one of the sites where oestrogen is produced. So, a little bit of weight gain around the waist is not necessarily a bad thing.

Strategies used in the past to lose weight may not work as well for either of you now. Calorie controlled diets are not the answer. Diets make your body think that you are being starved and as soon as you eat 'normally' again, it will replenish the fat stores in case there is a famine again! A better approach is about a long-term, different relationship with food.

It can be useful to keep a Food Journal to help identify any harmful eating patterns. You can download a journal at www.hotwomencoolsolutions.com.

Apples vs. Pears

The first sign of the start of perimenopause for some women may be gaining weight around the waist and changing to an 'apple' shape. Alternatively, they may put weight on around their hips and thighs giving rise to the 'pear' shape.

As explained above, a small amount of weight gain around the middle is ok. However excessive fat in that area can be a sign of stress and can be dangerous for health and particularly the risk of breast cancer (Glenville, 2006).

If your partner has started to become apple shaped, the time to take action is if the waist to hip ratio exceeds 0.8. To calculate this, measure her waist and hips and then divide the waist by the hip measurement. If the ratio is higher than 0.8 it can increase the risk of a range of conditions including cancer, high blood pressure, and stroke.

The 'Mindful Eating' advice below applies to 'Apples' and 'Pears'. For more advice on losing weight around the waist see *Fat Around the Middle* by Marilyn Glenville.

Underweight

This is not about being naturally slim or thin, this is about your partner's weight being too low to support her health and wellbeing. Being underweight is an issue at any stage of a woman's life. When younger women are underweight it can affect their periods and fertility. During perimenopause it can increase the risk of osteoporosis.

If your partner is generally eating well and they are losing weight they should seek advice from their doctor. It can be a sign of an overactive thyroid or celiac disease.

Mindful Eating

If you or your partner wants to lose weight or maintain a healthy weight, the first step is to understand the difference between physical and emotional hunger and only eat when you are physically hungry.

 There are two hormones that play an important role in regulating appetite and weight, ghrelin and leptin.

Ghrelin is produced by the stomach and sends the message that you need to eat. Ghrelin levels fall when the food you eat arrives at your intestines. If you go on an extreme diet, more ghrelin gets secreted and your ability to burn calories starts to diminish.

Leptin is a hormone secreted by fat cells which regulates appetite and metabolism. Levels of leptin rise as we eat so that the appetite is suppressed. It also promotes calorie burning.

The levels of leptin and ghrelin can also be affected by your sleep patterns. Studies have found that people who regularly slept for just five hours a night had 15 percent more ghrelin in their system, leading to feelings of hunger. They also had significantly less leptin to suppress the appetite. In light of this

> *research, it is important to sort out any sleep issues before you try to lose weight (see Chapter 4).*

Physical hunger comes on slowly. You might initially experience a loss of energy and concentration. This could be followed by irritability, light-headedness, a feeling of emptiness, hunger pangs and a strong desire to eat immediately. If you eat something when you are physically hungry, the hunger indicators will gradually fade away.

Emotional hunger comes on suddenly. You might start to salivate because you saw or smelled food. The urge to search the cupboards may also be motivated by feelings of sadness, anger, frustration—or most common of all—boredom. If you eat when you are emotionally hungry, you are likely to feel unsatisfied and possibly even sick.

If you start to eat before you're physically hungry you won't know when to stop eating. Also if you do not eat when you start to feel hungry you are more likely to crave carbohydrates. When you are starving hungry, a salad doesn't look like that appealing whereas a baguette or a sticky bun looks just right. Therefore being aware of your current level of hunger is important.

The signals for thirst and hunger are very similar so if you start to feel hungry, have a drink of water and then wait for ten minutes to feel if the hunger signal is still there. If it is, go ahead and eat.

The second step to losing or maintaining weight is to stop eating when you are satisfied. Do not wait for the 'full' or 'stuffed' signal as you will have eaten too much.

The secret to recognising these signals and having time to react to them is to eat mindfully, that is:

- Sit down when you eat—even if it's only a snack.
- Take time to enjoy your food—look at, smell, and taste the food.
- Slow down—put the knife and fork down between mouthfuls.
- Chew your food completely.
- Drink before you eat—don't drink while you are eating.
- Concentrate on eating—don't do anything but eat i.e. no TV, radio, or reading.
- Eat three meals a day—it is easier to keep track of your food intake if you eat regular meals rather than 'grazing'.

Right Foods

There is plenty of expert diet and nutrition advice available but the frustrating thing is that so much of it is contradictory. We accept the government's advice about having five portions of fruit and vegetables a day but other countries recommend seven portions and some as many as nine portions!

You can gain weight on any food and you can lose weight on any food so eat things that you enjoy but only eat between the levels of hunger and satisfaction. If you find it hard to leave food on the plate at the end of a meal, and many people do, take care with your portion size. Your body only wants about a fist size portion of food at any one feeding. By tuning into the signals coming from your stomach what you want to eat and what your body most wants to eat will gradually converge.

By eating solid proteins, such as lean meats and nuts, the level of ghrelin in your system stays lower and you feel fuller longer. If you eat simple sugars and carbohydrates the level of ghrelin will spike and you will feel hungry again quickly.

There are also lots of food myths to be beware of. For example there is the myth that fat free food is calorie free. In fact 'Low Fat' and 'Fat Free' foods are often higher in sugars and chemicals added in attempts to restore flavour. Therefore they can be more fattening and less nutritious than regular food. It is always a good idea to check food labels.

If you are eating out at a fast food restaurant many of them offer a 'healthy option' but beware. A 2005 report found that five out of eight salads sold by McDonalds,

Burger King, KFC, and Pizza Hut had high salt or fat content. For example one Big Mac has 540 calories and 1040 mg of salt; one premium southwest salad with crispy chicken and dressing has 530 calories and 1,260 mg of salt.

The lesson from all this is that it is better to eat simple, unprocessed foods whenever possible so that you know exactly what you are eating.

Some general food guidelines:

- Start the day with breakfast—people who do find it easier to lose weight. Eating protein at breakfast will keep you feeling fuller for longer.
- Keep your diet healthy, balanced, and satisfying.
- Soup stays longer in the stomach and delays hunger pangs.
- Eat vegetables that grow above ground—they store less sugar.
- Watch your portion size—reducing the size of your plate will reduce your food intake.
- Don't skip meals. If you let yourself get too hungry you will want to eat carbohydrates.

Eating out can be a real challenge when you are establishing new eating habits and trying to lose weight. When you are eating socially what's important isn't the food—it's the company. The problem is that when you are chatting with your friends you can lose track of what you are eating and how you are eating it. A few alcoholic drinks not only add calories they also make you less aware of the food.

Whether you are eating in a restaurant or at a dinner party keep to the same guidelines for mindful eating i.e., eat slowly and stop eating as soon as you are satisfied. Some more tips:

- Push the bread basket away and resist the temptation to eat before your meal starts by sipping water and chatting with your companions. If the bread rolls are served by a waiter just smile and say "Not for me, thank you".
- Don't over order or overload your plate. You may be able to order two starters instead of a starter and a main course.
- You don't have to eat everything on your plate. If it really upsets you to leave food on your plate in a restaurant ask for a doggie bag. At dinner parties just say "That was great, I'm really full."
- Ask for sauce or gravy on the side so that you can have a smaller amount.
- Trade potatoes for an extra vegetable that you enjoy.
- If you want a desert, share one with a friend.

Alcohol can be an issue if your partner is experiencing hot flashes. There's no reason why women can't enjoy a drink (unless otherwise advised by their doctor) so long as they drink in moderation and make sensible choices. Weight for weight, alcohol contains more calories than sugar, so even moderate drinking can lead to weight gain.

Establishing new eating habits and a new relationship to food can take time and there will be days when it is difficult. But if you and your partner keep going back to the guidelines they will just become how you normally eat and you won't have to think about them anymore. This is not an 'all or nothing' approach.

Food Supplements

If you or your partner wants to lose weight there are supplements that claim to help your body burn off excess fat and reduce stress hormones. These weight-related supplements typically contain one or more of the following:

Chromium—to control insulin levels

B vitamins—for glucose metabolism and to balance blood sugar

Magnesium—for the calming effect on the body

Zinc—to aid the production of hormones, including leptin

Vitamin C—to regulate blood sugar

Omega-3 fats—to help burn off fat

All supplements should be used as directed and in conjunction with the healthier approach to eating outlined above. There is more information about food supplements in the Resources section.

Exercise

When you are trying to lose or maintain weight you are often given the 'eat less, exercise more' or the 'calories in, calories burnt' message but the science behind this is a lot less straightforward than it seems (Harcombe, 2011).

What is undisputable is that exercise is good for your mental and physical wellbeing. Exercise will speed up your metabolism which will help to burn off calories. This does not mean that you need to sign up for the gym. There are plenty of additional activities and exercises that you can do at home (see Chapter 7).

Be aware that if you do additional exercise you may start to believe that you can eat more. During and after exercise, drink plenty of water so that you lessen the hunger signal. Don't reward yourself with food for exercise.

If you have any weight-related health issues or your body mass index (BMI) is over 30 you should consult your Doctor before you start doing regular exercise. You can calculate your BMI by going to:

http://www.nhs.uk/Tools/Pages/Healthyweightcalculator .aspx?r=1&rtitle=Interactive+tools+-+BMI+tool and entering your details.

Your Bonus

You can download a relaxation/hypnotic recording to help to support your weight loss at www.hotwomencoolsolutions.com.

CHAPTER 6

HOW DO WE REVITALISE OUR RELATIONSHIP IN THE BEDROOM?

"My wife and I are experiencing a new phase in our lives where we can enjoy sex, have fun with it, try out new things and be relaxed. We have experimented with lots of different positions and had sex in some different places which adds to the fun and overall excitement.

"At times I think my wife has been a bit self-conscious about her body but I keep telling her that my body is changing too. I am pleased to say that we are both healthy and we exercise regularly to keep ourselves in shape. I think my wife is sexy and I am happy to tell her so!"

This stage of your life could be the best time for your sex life with your hot woman. The sex may be as whizz bang as it has always been but slower. It can also be more sensitive and intense. You both have more experience now and you have learned more along the way. You may not have to wait for the children to go to sleep or worry about interruptions any more. This can be a time for exploring and enjoying without the worry of contraception.

There can be a perception that the changes to the hormones during perimenopause lead to a reduction in libido but actually they can lead to heightened sexual response. Responses from older women in the Hite Report support this:

"I didn't know getting older would make sex better! I'm fifty-one now and just getting started."

"I thought that menopause was the leading factor in my dry and irritable vaginal tract. My doctors thought that it was lack of hormones . . . but with my new lover, I am reborn. Plenty of lubrication, no irritation."

A study in 1986 (Masters & Johnson) found that women have no decline in orgasmic potential during their lives and may become more orgasmic.

If your partner is already going through perimenopause and has noticed a reduction in sex drive think about what might be contributing to it. Factors that might contribute to a reduced sex drive are:

- Tiredness
- Stress
- Too much alcohol
- Depression
- Low-thyroid function

A factor that has an enormous influence on sex drive during later life is beliefs. If your partner believes that sexiness belongs to the young, thin, and perfect women that you see every day on TV and in adverts then the chances are that they won't believe they measure up to it. However if they believe that being sexy is about how confident they feel and the chemistry between the two of you then you are more likely to carry on with a healthy and confident sex life long past menopause.

Sex

Sex is good for men and women. It's not just about the enjoyment; sex stimulates the hormones, releases tension, boosts the immune system, relieves headaches, and is a great form of exercise. A research project involving 55,000 respondents showed that people who had a satisfying sex life were physically healthier and more relaxed than those with an unsatisfying sex life (Institute for Advanced Study of Human Sexuality, San Francisco).

This is not only about penetrative sex. There is a whole range of foreplay and intimate touch that will stimulate the production of positive hormones, improve your mood and tone your body.

You can get back in touch each other's bodies through massage. Massage is always sensual and does not have to be the precursor to sex if you don't want it to be. It can be a way of finding out more about what parts of the body are particularly sensuous for you and your partner. You can experiment with different types of oil and creams and lubricants and with different textures to heighten the experience for example feathers, fur, and ice.

Relationships

Communication is essential to the success of your relationship generally and your sexual relationship in particular. There needs to be an understanding of each other's needs.

If you are in a long-term relationship, sex may be a subject that you have stopped talking about. You may think that you know what your partner is thinking about you and your relationship but the chances are that if you haven't talked about it recently, you do not know what they really think. If you are at the beginning of a new relationship, now is the chance to be open and honest about what you enjoy.

So, how do you start that conversation? It's probably not a good idea to have the conversation in bed when you are both feeling tired or under pressure. Think about having a chat away from your everyday situation. You could arrange to have a date for example. Be imaginative, it doesn't have to be going out for a meal, you could have a trip to a spa so that you could both relax and have a massage or other treatment.

Once you understand each other better you can explore what works best for both of you. You might consider visiting a shop that sells lingerie and sex toys. Staff in these shops are trained to assist you and they won't be embarrassed so you don't need to be either. If you don't feel that confident you can always shop for what you want on the Internet.

Pregnancy

Women can get pregnant during the perimenopause. HRT does not act as contraception and, because your partner may still be ovulating when she first starts taking it, she could get pregnant. As a general guideline, you should wait for two clear years after her last period before you stop using contraception.

If you are in a new relationship, use a barrier method such as condoms because of the risk of sexually transmitted diseases.

Incontinence

What woman wants to talk to her partner about incontinence? Incontinence, or the involuntary loss of control of the bladder, is an embarrassing problem that can affect women at any age regardless of whether they have given birth or not. A third of all women suffer bladder control problems (Chiarelli, 1995).

Incontinence comes in two types:

- Urge incontinence—a sudden need to urinate and not being able to get to the toilet in time.
- Stress incontinence—is the most common form of incontinence. It often leads to urinating while sneezing, laughing, or exercising. At menopause it can arise from pelvic floor issues. The pelvic floor is a complex group of muscles that is generally poorly understood but strengthening them will assist with bladder control and improve the experience of sex.

Pelvic floor exercises, known as Kegels, can be started at any age and if your partner is already experiencing menopause symptoms it's definitely a case of 'better late than never'. For more information and exercises see the Resources Section

If pelvic floor exercises do not improve your partner's symptoms or the problem persists there may be some underlying cause that needs further investigation.

Encourage her to consult her doctor about medication and treatment options.

Languages of love

You may feel like you are doing and saying everything right but you are still not achieving a good response from your partner it may be that you are not using the correct 'language'. In his best-selling book, *The Five Love Languages*, Dr Gary Chapman suggests that we all express love to others in a way that would make us feel loved. But that may not be the way that makes your partner feel loved. Dr Chapman states that the five love languages are:

1. Words of affirmation—these could be words of praise, encouragement, or kindness such: "That's a great idea", "Well done", "Thank you so much for . . .", "I am so proud of the way you . . ."
2. Gifts—a gift does not have to be big or expensive, it just has to express love. It could be related to a particular interest the other person has, or something they have mentioned, or something that enhances their life.
3. Acts of service—this could be as small as taking a cup of tea to your partner, or loading the dishwasher, up to solving a problem for the other person such as arranging to take her parents for a hospital appointment.
4. Quality time—the most basic type of quality time is listening to your partner. It can also be

taking part in their interests or taking part in a joint activity such as a going out for a meal or taking a holiday.

5. Physical touch—this is not just about sex, it's also about loving touch, hugs, cuddles, and hand-holding.

First understand your own love language by observing your own reactions and noticing what makes you feel loved. Then start to observe your partner. Notice their expressions, their complaints, and their requests. If you partner sits next to you to watch TV and pulls your arm around their shoulders you can guess that they are looking for physical touch. If they say, "Can we go for a walk together?" then they are looking for quality time. You get the idea.

Discovering your partner's language may take a bit of time and effort but it will be rewarding for your relationship.

CHAPTER 7

HOW CAN WE BOTH STAY FIT AND HEALTHY?

"We made a decision a couple of years ago to get more exercise. We had both put on a bit of weight and I am on medication for high blood pressure and high cholesterol. Neither of us plays any sports so we decided to join our local gym which also has a swimming pool.

"We try to go to the gym twice a week and we generally succeed. I use a combination of the cardiovascular machines such as the running-machine and the cross-trainer plus some of the weights machines. My wife mainly uses the car-diovascular machines and sometimes goes swimming.

"We both feel better for it and it is keeping our weight under control." Tom

Health issues

If men and women go into their middle years in a fit and healthy condition, there is no reason why they can't come out of the other side of it just as fit and healthy. Some of the health issues associated with menopause are more likely to be related to getting older or lifestyle issues and these can affect men as well as women.

There are some health issues that are specifically related to the physical changes that are linked to the hormonal changes of the menopause.

Heart Disease

The terms cardiovascular or heart disease are general terms that can cover angina, heart attack, stroke, coronary artery disease, and high blood pressure. Heart disease is the UK's biggest killer of women. Women are twice as likely to die from heart disease as any form of cancer.

Prior to menopause, oestrogen helps to protect the heart by balancing levels of 'good' (HDL) and 'bad' (LDL) cholesterol and keeping blood vessels healthy. Because of this there is a higher risk of heart disease post menopause.

If there is a family history of heart disease or stroke you and your partner may have an increased risk of developing heart disease. But you are not a victim of your genes. There are various lifestyle choices that impact on the risk of heart disease including weight, exercise, smoking, drinking alcohol, and stress.

Hypertension

Hypertension is the medical name for high blood pressure and becomes more likely with age. You are said to have hypertension when your blood pressure reading is consistently in excess of 140/90 mm Hg. It affects nearly 30 percent of people worldwide and is a frequent cause of strokes and heart attacks.

There are two types of hypertension. Primary (or essential) hypertension is the term used for high blood pressure that has no known cause and over 90 percent of cases are in this category. Secondary hypertension refers to high blood pressure that is the result of a disease or other medically recognised cause, for example sleep apnea, kidney disease, excess cortisol, or other hormone disorders.

Common symptoms of high blood pressure are headaches, blurred vision, nosebleeds, tinnitus (buzzing in the ears), and dizziness. If you or your partner has any of these symptoms and you think you might have high blood pressure you may be able to have it checked at your local pharmacy. If

> *you are still concerned go to see your medical practitioner who may prescribe medication and give you dietary and lifestyle advice. The sooner it is treated the better.*

There are actions that you can both take to reduce your risk of high blood pressure in addition to taking medication. Common diet and lifestyle issues that aggravate your blood pressure are:

- Salt—Reduce salt in your diet by not adding salt when cooking and eating, avoiding or limiting processed foods that contain added salt e.g., breakfast cereals, cakes and biscuits, and eating fresh or frozen vegetables. Check labels on processed foods for 'salt' or 'sodium'.
- Alcohol—Control your alcohol intake by drinking water to quench your thirst before and between alcoholic drinks, start drinking later in the day, and using a bottle stopper so that you don't feel compelled to finish the bottle.
- Exercise—Lack of exercise affects circulation, metabolism, and weight. If you are not used to exercise and you have high blood pressure you should start off slowly with small exercise goals and build up. See below for more advice. *
- Excess weight—See Chapter 5.
- Stress—Reduce stress by finding a method of relaxation you enjoy such as meditation, yoga, or walking. See Chapter 6.

- Smoking—The incidence of hypertension rises if you smoke 15 or more cigarettes a day. Women who smoke are more at risk of heart attack, stroke, and peripheral vascular disease. The advice is simple—stop smoking!

Breast Health

As women enter perimenopause they may notice changes to the size, shape, and firmness of their breasts. There may also be changes to the size and sensitivity of their nipples.

Tender and sore breasts can cause some discomfort. At night, heating pads, warm water bottles, and lavender oil mixed with a carrier oil may alleviate discomfort. It is important to wear a properly fitted bra that supports the breasts, preferably without underwires.

However, the main issue for women as they enter their forties and fifties is the risk of breast cancer. The incidence of breast cancer rises with age. Having a family history of breast cancer, especially among close female relatives, can increase the risk but only 5-10 per cent of cases are due to genetic predisposition. Other risk factors include:

- Early onset of menstruation and a late menopause
- Having children later than average (e.g., after age thirty-five)

- Obesity
- A diet high in sugars and animal or dairy fat

Although breast cancer is often thought of as a disease that only affects women it can also affect men. It affects just one in every 100,000 men in England, mainly over seventy years of age. The causes of breast cancer in men are similar to those for women. The common symptoms of breast cancer in men are:

- A hard painless lump in one breast
- Hard, inflamed and sore nipples
- The nipple turning in on itself
- Fluid leaking from the nipple

The good news is that nearly 40 percent of breast cancers could be prevented by maintaining a healthy body weight, reducing alcohol intake, exercising regularly, eating less red meat, and eating more fruit and vegetables.

In the UK, breast screening is recommended for women between the ages of fifty and seventy. A mammogram is an x-ray carried out by compressing the breasts between two plates. It is an uncomfortable process and can be quite painful but it is over quickly and can provide an early indication of cancer.

It is important to carry out regular monthly breast examinations to check for lumps or irregularities. The indicators to look for include small lumps, dimples or dents in the skin when lifting your arm, reddish, ulcerated or scaly skin on the breasts or nipples, any bleeding or discharge from the nipple, or any change in nipple position i.e., pulled inwards or pointing in a different direction.

Encourage your partner to check her breasts by following the steps below:

1. Stand in front of the mirror with your top half naked. Have your arms by your side.
2. Raise your arms and put your hands behind your head. Look for differences in the shape or texture of the breasts and the nipples. Check for discharge.
3. Lie down with your head and shoulders on a pillow. Lift your right arm and put your hand behind your head. Using your left hand with the fingers flat, stroke the right breast and underarm using gentle circular motions. Note any changes or irregularities
4. Repeat for the left breast.

If you or your partner notices anything that concerns you, go to see your medical practitioner as soon as possible. Most breast problems are benign, not cancerous, and early diagnosis and treatment leads to better results.

Heavy Bleeding

In the pre-menopause stage, your partner may notice a change in her menstrual flow. It can vary in length and in volume between very light to heavy and flooding. The major cause of heavy menstrual bleeding is the variation in the levels of progesterone.

If your partner experiences frequent, very heavy bleeding (menorrhagia) over a prolonged period of time, she needs to consult her medical practitioner. Heavy bleeding can be caused by fibroids, endometriosis, pelvic inflammatory disease, and uterine or cervical cancer.

Heavy periods can leave a woman feeling exhausted and drained. They can also result in iron deficiency anaemia and she may need to take an iron supplement. Symptoms of anaemia include feeling tired, dizziness, shortness of breath, sore tongue, and headaches. Use an organic iron supplement as it is easier to absorb and less likely to cause constipation than ferrous sulphate. Take vitamin C with the iron supplement as it is essential for absorption. Vitamin A may also be beneficial.

There are changes that can be made to diet to help to control heavy bleeding. Reducing the amount of meat and dairy products and increasing the intake of essential fatty acids (for example linseed oil) may help with this issue.

A woman experiencing heavy bleeding also needs to increase her intake of water and non-caffeinated drinks to stay hydrated.

Osteoporosis

Osteoporosis literally means 'porous bones'. The clinical definition is 'a condition where there is less normal bone than expected for a woman's age, with an increased risk of fracture'. It can affect both men and women.

Osteoporosis isn't painful and most people don't realise that they have it until they fracture a bone after a relatively minor accident or stress. One visible sign of osteoporosis is the characteristic bending forward position that develops in older people.

The bone mass of both men and women reduce naturally as they get older but women are more likely to develop osteoporosis. In women in the perimenopause stage, the risk of developing the condition is partly due to the reduction in the levels of oestrogen but there are other important factors involved.

Genetics is a factor. If your partner has a mother or father with osteoporosis they may be at higher risk of developing the condition. Women are more at risk it they have an early menopause (before age forty-five) or their menstrual periods are absent for more than six months due to over-exercising or over-dieting. Some medications can affect bone density.

However, as with the other health issues already discussed, diet and lifestyle can weaken or strengthen your bones. In addition to the guidance given above for dealing with hypertension there are other changes that can be made specifically to keep bones strong:

- Resistance exercise—for example weight training at the gym, using resistance bands, or doing household and gardening tasks that involve lifting.
- Alkaline diet—eat more alkaline fruit, vegetables, eggs, and fish.
- Limit caffeine, sugar, alcohol, and fizzy drinks.
- Reduce refined bran. Eat bran as part of the whole grain for example oats or brown rice.
- Food supplements—calcium and vitamin D are important for bone health. Vitamin B is also recommended (Glenville, 2011).

If you or your partner is at high risk for osteoporosis your doctor may refer you for a bone density scan which is known as a DEXA scan. This painless procedure measures your bone mineral density and compares it to the bone density of a healthy young adult and someone who is the same age and sex as you. If the results indicate osteoporosis, your doctor may prescribe drugs (bisphosphonates, strontium ranelate, calcitonin, or HRT) and give you advice on food supplements, diet, and life-style.

Headaches and Migraine

There is a big difference between headaches and migraines, as you will know if you have experienced the latter. Headaches are painful but not usually associated with other symptoms. Migraines can be associated with a range of other symptoms including blurring and changes in vision, fatigue, nausea, and vomiting.

Some women experience migraines at the beginning of their menstrual cycle and as they reach menopause these migraines stop. Other women have migraines at ovulation or during the second half of the menstrual cycle due to insufficient amounts of progesterone being produced at this time. The same imbalance can occur during perimenopause. Migraine can also be a side effect of HRT.

Some types of food and drink can contribute to headaches for example cheese, chocolate, onions, caffeine, and alcohol.

Headaches can also be related to sleep problems and stress (see Chapter 9).

Meditation, yoga, and relaxation exercises can help to ease headaches. Some people also get relief from a hot bath with essential oils such as melissa or lavender.

There are a number of over-the-counter painkillers that can ease headaches in the short term.

If you or your partner is suffering from acute or persistent migraines it is important to consult your health care practitioner to confirm that you do not have an underlying health issue.

Constipation

Constipation is defined as having a bowel movement fewer than three times a week. Some people with constipation find it painful to have a bowel movement and experience bloating and the sensation of a full bowel.

Some women experience constipation during the menopause due to a lack of progesterone. This reduces the movement of food through the intestines so that bowel movements become infrequent, dry, and pebble-like.

There are some common foods that can dry out stools and aggravate constipation. These include potatoes, puffed cereals, and toast. Apples and pears can clog your system and should be eaten baked or steamed. Dried fruit should be soaked and rinsed before eating.

Some medications including pain medications, antacids, and blood pressure treatments can cause constipation. So if you are experiencing constipation, check the side effects of any medications that you are taking.

Sometimes all you need to relieve constipation is just to drink more fluids and eat more fibre. You need to drink approximately six to eight glasses of water or non-caffeine drinks a day. Good sources of fibre are fruit, vegetables, and whole grains.

Physical activity helps to keep food flowing through the body effectively. Regular exercise that includes cardiovascular and weight training activity will be most effective.

Exercise

A recent worldwide study concluded that lack of exercise is more harmful than smoking in terms of your risk of developing chronic diseases (The Lancet, 2012). Exercise is anything that causes you to breathe more deeply than you normally would or causes your heart rate to speed up. Fitness is the ability to perform physical activity.

Exercise is good for your physical, mental, and emotional health. It can help you to maintain a healthy weight and reduce the risk Alzheimer's disease associated with obesity. It improves your posture, making you look younger

Research carried out in Australia found that women in the age range 45–60 who exercised two or more times a week reported fewer headaches, felt less tense, tired, and fatigued, and had lower rates of mental symptoms of depression than non-exercisers (Ratey and Hagerman, 2009).

How much exercise?

To control weight and ease menopause symptoms it is good to have some form of aerobic exercise four days a week. If you are starting from a level of no exercise, this may seem daunting but the important thing is to get into a routine so that after a few weeks it just becomes part of what you do and you hardly notice that you are doing it.

The most effective exercise programme is to have a mix of cardio-vascular activity that raises your heart rate, and resistance exercise (e.g., using weights or resistance bands) to protect your bones against osteoporosis and maintain your upper body strength and muscle tone.

For cardio vascular activity (e.g., walking, jogging, swimming etc), you want to aim to raise your pulse up to 60 or 65 percent of your maximum heart rate and keep it there for about an hour.

Some General Guidelines

- Set realistic, specific goals, plan to achieve them, and take action.
- Two 10 minute bursts of exercise every day or 30 minutes four days a week will make a difference.
- Drink plenty of water before and after exercise.
- Vary your exercise and pick activities you enjoy.
- Wait at least two hours after eating before vigorous exercise.
- Don't exercise if you feel unwell.
- If you have chest pains, dizziness, or excessive shortness of breath, stop exercising immediately.

Exercise suggestions

Planned exercise:

Dancing	Netball	Yoga	Pilates
Football	Tennis	Badminton	Squash
Aquacise	Circuit training	Walking	Jogging
Athletics	Skipping	Boxing	Weight training
Gym	Zumba	Aerobics	Step classes
Spin classes	Rugby	Sailing	Swimming

Opportunistic exercise:

Around the home

- Gardening—a bit of digging can burn off 150 cal in half an hour.
- Stairs—running up and down the stairs 10 times a day will burn off 250 cal and tone the thighs.
- Housework—ironing 150 cal in half an hour; vacuuming 200 cal in half an hour.
- Sex—30 minutes of sex-ercise will burn off 200 cal and tone stomach muscles and inner thighs.

At the office

- Park the car further from the office and walk.
- Ditch the elevator and take the stairs.
- Walk to deliver messages rather than emailing or phoning.

Shopping

- Park as far away from the shop entrance as possible.
- Carry purchases to the car to burn off more calories.

Walking

Walking is excellent exercise because it costs nothing and there are lots of opportunities to enjoy it every day.

You can burn off significant calories through walking and it is good for strengthening your lungs and heart.

For more information about walking and calorie calculators see www.walking.about.com.

CHAPTER 8

WHAT CAN WE DO TO KEEP OUR MINDS HEALTHY?

"I have noticed that my wife is more easily stressed since she started going through her menopause. She has always been decisive but now she seems to have problems making decisions. I wonder if it is caused by lack of sleep because she has hot flashes during the night that disturb her sleep—and mine!

"She has a demanding job and we are still supporting our youngest son financially and emotionally. I think she is just tired most of the time." Peter

Just as you may be noticing physical changes in you and your partner during this stage, you may also notice mental and emotional changes. Changes to the cognitive ability of men and women as they enter their fifties can be due to brain shrinkage that occurs naturally due to loss of water content.

Research has shown that verbal memory can be affected by fluctuating oestrogen levels. Oestrogen's relationship to memory and language relates to how the brain stores information. Some women find that they forget common words or have problems with reading during the menopause.

Fluctuating hormone levels can also contribute to less efficient cognitive functions but most of these symptoms are relatively mild and transient. So, you may find yourself forgetting words or walking to the top of the stairs and forgetting why you are there but you can minimise these effects by keeping your brain healthy and lively.

If you or your partner thinks that your memory loss is more severe than this, you should consult your doctor. Indicators to be aware of are:

- Disorientation in familiar surroundings
- Inability to remember recent conversations
- Trouble making decisions
- Repeating stories in the same conversation
- Confusion with simple tasks
- Trouble learning something new
- Trouble counting money.

Can hormone replacement therapy help with memory?

As the production of oestrogen and progesterone starts to falter during perimenopause, the brain's delicate balance of neurochemicals gets disrupted.

At one time it was believed that hormone replacement therapy could help prevent dementia, memory loss, and Alzheimer's disease but research no longer appears to support this. A British study reported that women on HRT have twice the risk of developing dementia.

There are studies that support the use of HRT for short periods during menopause. A study by the University of Illinois published in 2005 showed that women who took HRT for ten years or less had greater brain volume than women who had never taken it or those who had taken it for more than ten years. In the same study, the women were tested for aerobic fitness and when those results were factored in, it was shown that exercise and fitness had a significant positive effect on measures of performance and brain volume.

If your partner is considering taking HRT it is important to discuss all of the benefits and the risks with a doctor.

Exercise Your Mind

I have already talked about the benefits of physical exercise on maintaining cognitive ability. There are also mental exercises that you can do to keep you sharp. It could be doing quizzes, crosswords, or puzzles every day, or you could try some of the following suggestions:

1) Make changes in the location of frequently used objects in your home or office. If you have to think about where you have put your tea bags, or favourite pen, or hair brush it will help you to set up new neural pathways. You could just try using your other hand to move your mouse or brush your teeth.

2) Make changes to your daily routine for the same reason as 1) above.

3) Decide to learn something new every day/week/ month. This can be something small like learning a new word every day to something big like enrolling for an evening class or taking up a new hobby.

4) Try using one of the computer-based brain exercises such as MindFit or Brain Gym.

Whatever you decide to do, you need to do it regularly—after all you don't get good at jogging by going for one run.

There are many different exercises that you can do to improve your memory and I have included some links in the Resources section. Neuroscientists have given us some good tips recently for those moments of forgetfulness:

- If you go somewhere to get something and then forget what it was, go back to the room you started in and try again. Apparently, physical doorways act as memory thresholds and you stand a better chance of remembering if you are in the location where you had the initial thought.
- If you can't remember where you put something say out loud the name of the item several times. This primes your unconscious to find the object.

The Time of Your Life

This stage in the lives of you and your partner can be one of changes in many areas:

- **Relationships**—you may be facing the challenges of a long-term relationship or a new relationship.
- **Children**—teenage children can pose all sorts of issues or you may be experiencing an 'empty nest'.

- **Parents**—you may find yourself dealing with elderly parents at the same time as supporting your growing children.
- **Work**—you may have reached a more demanding level in your career or be thinking about doing something new.
- **Finances**—this may be a time when you are starting to notice your finances easing or facing the demands of supporting children going off to university or at home without jobs.

Any or all of these changes can be a challenge that you can deal with and learn from but if there is too much pressure you may both experience stress. Stress can be defined as a state we experience when perceived demands exceed perceived ability to cope. This mismatch can give rise to positive feelings of stretch or stress depending on the nature of the imbalance.

Stress arises when you are faced with an increase in demand and the mind perceives that the resources available are insufficient to meet these. A series of nervous and hormonal processes are set into action, resulting in what is commonly described as the fight or flight response.

There is a wide variety of symptoms associated with stress. You might experience:

- PHYSICAL SYMPTOMS—headaches, sweaty palms, sleeping problems, dizziness, back pain, neck and shoulder pain, palpitations, weight gain around the waist, and increased infections like colds and flu

- BEHAVIOURAL SYMPTOMS—increased cig–arette smoking, alcohol intake, or a decrease or increase in your appetite may cause you to have difficulty relaxing and find that you lose your temper more easily.
- EMOTIONAL SYMPTOMS—crying, edginess, anger, worries about health, and mood swings
- COGNITIVE AND MENTAL SYMPTOMS—trouble concentrating, memory problems, inability to make decisions, and loss of a sense of humour

Stress could also affect your work performance through absenteeism, poor time keeping, overworking, a decline in your usual standards, sloppy work, or being more irritable with colleagues.

It is important to be able to manage your stress because our bodies have not evolved to deal with sustained high levels of stress and it increases your risk of a range of life threatening illnesses including heart disease and cancer.

Emotional Resilience

Emotional resilience refers to the ability to spring back emotionally after you have experienced a difficult or stressful time in your life. People who are emotionally resilient are able to recover quickly from the effects of powerful negative emotions such as anger, anxiety, and depression. They are more able to keep problems in perspective and are not easily overwhelmed.

There are certain attitudes and behaviours that make people more emotionally resilient. Some people seem to be born with these attitudes but if that's not you, you can develop them.

Emotional Resilience Trait	How to develop it
Acknowledging how you feel and why—you have a right to your emotions without letting them take over your life	1 Notice your negative thoughts and how they are influencing your emotions (see Faulty Thinking in Chapter 4)
	2 Wear a rubber band on your wrist and when you notice a negative thought arising, twang the band and tell yourself to 'Stop it!'
	3 Develop positive self-talk—every morning look in the mirror, smile, and repeat a positive affirmation to yourself for example 'I am feeling calmer/more confident/ stronger every day.'

Understanding how much control you have over your life—believing that the actions you take contribute to better outcomes influences how you respond to stress in a positive manner	Recognise that you always have options. In any situation you can look for opportunities to: i) **Avoid** the people or situations that stress you. ii) **Alter** the situation so that it is more acceptable. iii) **Adapt** by taking a more positive approach, adjusting your standards, or looking at the 'big picture'. iv) **Accept** and don't try to control the uncontrollable. Learn to forgive. Evaluate each option and decide on the best.
Being optimistic—being able to view the world in an optimistic light allows you to develop your strengths and resources	1 Live a healthy lifestyle. 2 Set yourself achievable goals. 3 Celebrate your successes. 4 Don't beat yourself up about the things that don't go right. There is no failure—only feedback. 5 Spend some time picturing the positive future that you want to achieve and plan to achieve it.

Having social contacts – those with strong social networks tend to stay happier and healthier and cope better with challenges and stress	There are lots of opportunities to build your social network: 1 Join a sports club or exercise class. 2 Enrol for an evening class or day school for a subject you are interested in. 3 Get involved in a hobby group. 4 Contact your friends and arrange a get together.
Enjoying a laugh—laughing at life's adversities helps to immunise you against stress.	1 Put coloured stickers around your home and undertake to smile whenever you spot one. 2 Put aside time to have a laugh every day. Have a selection of funny books and videos to choose from. 3 Call a friend who you know makes you laugh. 4 Join a laughter therapy group
Exercising—exercise releases positive hormones into the blood and reinforces the message to your unconscious that you are looking after yourself.	All exercise is good for your physical and emotional health. To feel calmer you could try yoga or tai chi. Walking and talking with a friend is good exercise that you hardly notice.

Connecting with your environment—noticing the things of nature around you helps you to keep problems in perspective.	Take time each day to notice the things of nature around you. Go for a walk and just look around.
Caring for others—random acts of kindness to others is good for them and can make you happier.	1 Decide to commit a random act of kindness every day. Could be as small as a smile to a shop worker or a compliment to a colleague. 2 Volunteer. Get involved with a charity or group or your local church.

Supplements

There is frequently debate in the media about whether you need to take food supplements to stay emotionally healthy. The argument is generally around whether you can get all of the nutrients you need from a well-balanced diet.

If you are experiencing some of the symptoms of stress it may be helpful to support your system with supplements. You could consider taking daily multivitamins with minerals, vitamin C, and omega-3 fish oil capsules.

Physical Exercise

Exercise is important to your mental and emotional health as well as your physical health. It helps balance the effects of diminished hormones and can protect against cognitive decline. Exercise stimulates the production of neurotransmitters and neurotrophins and creates more receptors for them in key areas of the brain.

The University of Queensland, Australia surveyed 833 women between the ages of forty-five to sixty. They found that 84 percent of women questioned exercised two or more times a week and reported that they had significantly lower rates of the physical and mental symptoms of depression than non-exercisers. In particular they felt less tense, tired, and fatigued (Ratey, 2009).

Exercise is also important for your brain. One study showed that the most physical active women over the age of sixty-five had a 30 percent lower risk of cognitive decline. This was not dependent on the intensity of the exercise but on the amount.

In order to keep your brain healthy you need to do some aerobic exercise at least four days a week. That could be brisk walking, jogging, or any activity that raises your pulse rate to 60 or 65 percent of your maximum heart rate.

CHAPTER 9

HOW DO WE STAY HAPPY DURING ALL THIS CHANGE?

"This is my second marriage and I am a few years older than my wife. I am in my sixties and she is just entering her fifties and starting to experience menopause symptoms. Our daughters are still in their teens which can be challenging. At the same time, my wife's parents are elderly and starting to need regular support.

All of this is stressing my wife out and she is tearful and not sleeping well. I provide as much support as I can but I wish I could do more. I just want her to be happy."

Many clients come to me because they want to be happy but what does happy mean? You know happiness when you see it in other people.

Happy people tend to have an upright posture with their head up and shoulders down. They breathe lower in their chest and their eyes are level and alert. And, of course, they smile.

Happiness is very important to your health and well-being and laughter really is the best medicine. Laughter:

- Increases the disease fighting protein Gamma-interferon

- Increases T-cells and B-cells, which make disease fighting anti-bodies

- Benefits the heart

- Lowers blood pressure

- Lowers stress hormones

- Strengthens abdominal muscles

- Relaxes the body

- Reduces pain, possibly through the production of endorphins

Happier people even live longer!

There are certain key hormones that are associated with happiness:

- *Dopamine—the motivation chemical. It increases our ability to focus and motivates us to take action. Dopamine levels rise as we move towards a goal and begin to anticipate a result. Highest when we are in active pursuit of getting our most basic needs met.*
- *Serotonin—the feel good chemical. It is calming and soothing. Highest when we win anything, get public recognition for a job well done, or feel part of a crowd, group, or team.*
- *Endorphins—the body's natural pain killer. Can create euphoria. Endorphins are released when you exercise, make love, laugh a lot, or relax deeply. The presence of endorphins in the blood makes you feel better and can make you smarter.*
- *Noradrenaline—is synthesised from tyrosine. Noradrenaline can elevate mood.*
- *PEA (phenylethylamine)—produces a walking on air feeling. It is manufactured during vigorous exercise.*
- *Oxytocin—the 'love' hormone is associated with maternal bonding. Released when we kiss or hug someone affectionately*

What Causes Low Mood or Depression?

Depression can affect both men and women and it is not a symptom of menopause. I have included it here because you can experience it at this stage of your life possibly due to the effects of reduced levels of hormones combined with other life events. Although more women than men are diagnosed with depression the actual distribution by gender appears to be equal (Yapko, 1994).

There are various theories about the causes of depression. The biological theories concern the link between depression and the lack of certain chemicals in the brain. Also there is a link between depression and certain physical disorders such as substance abuse, heart disease, surgery, and diseases of the kidneys, liver, and lungs. (Hollister, 1983)

The 'Human Givens approach' suggests that depression arises when you experience unmet physical, psychological, or emotional needs such as the needs for shelter, safety, attention, privacy, and friendship. Unmet needs can arise from a major life event such as death of a loved one, job loss, or a serious medical problem.

If your needs are not met, you begin to worry about it, using your imagination to dwell on possible bad future situations. The mind/body does not differentiate between reality and imagination so it responds fearfully to both. The worries build up and this affects sleep which impacts on energy and motivation.

These thoughts and worries can be transient but if they persist for more than a month you should seek medical advice.

Common symptoms of clinical depression are:

- Feelings of hopelessness that lasts most of the day every day for two weeks or longer
- General tiredness and lack of energy
- Difficulty concentrating
- Loss of interest in activities that you have found pleasurable in the past
- Sleep disorder
- Self-harm
- Recurrent thoughts of suicide or death

Nutrition

There is a direct link between mood and blood sugar balance. Low blood sugar can lead to you feeling down and as though you have no energy. High blood sugar can leave you feeling so energised that you can't sit down.

To balance your blood sugar levels avoid sugary foods and refined carbohydrates such as white rice, white bread, and processed breakfast cereals. Reduce your intake of stimulants such as tea, coffee, chocolate, and cigarettes as these increase levels of the stress hormones adrenaline and cortisol, which also increase sugar levels.

Some food supplements may help to stabilise your mood:

- Chromium—stabilizes blood sugar levels.
- Omega-3 fish oils—increases levels of serotonin.
- B vitamins—people with low levels of folic acid are more likely to be depressed and less likely to get positive results from anti-depressant drugs.
- 5-HTP (amino acid 5-Hydroxy Tryptophan)—can be effective in treating depression. *Do not* take 5-HTP without your doctor's permission if you are currently taking anti-depressants.

Positive Worrying

As I have already said, people who are depressed worry a lot, often ruminating over their problems at night when they really want to go to sleep.

Worrying is not a bad thing in itself. It helps you to re–hearse future situations, assess risks, and plan for them. But when you are in a low mood you tend to only consider the worst case scenario—'Scary Street'! If you live on Scary Street long enough it will have a major impact on your mind/body system as it will release cortisol into your system and stress you out.

There is another way to think about the future. You can spend some time picturing the same event but with everything going well—that is 'Happy Valley'! This primes your brain for a positive outcome and releases the happiness hormones into your system.

Neither Scary Street or Happy Valley are real, they are just pictures of the future that you are constructing in your imagination. The only reality is the present moment.

A healthier way of worrying is to consider both possible outcomes.

1. Think about a future event/issue that you have concerns about.
2. Imagine the very worst outcome of that event. What are the risks connected to that event that could lead to it going wrong?
3. Imagine the very best outcome of that event. What actions could you take that would achieve that result?
4. What would be a realistic outcome between the best and the worst?

When you think about the worst case it is important to assess the level and likelihood of the risks occurring. If the worst possible outcome of the circumstance is life threatening and is likely to occur (e.g., if you don't wear a seat belt you are likely to be badly injured in a car accident) then you need to address that risk. If the risk you are worrying about is very unlikely to occur (e.g., aliens landing and disrupting your journey to an interview) stop thinking about it.

Mood Scale

I encourage clients who come to me because they are experiencing depression to be aware of their current mood level. It is useful in alerting them to take action to correct it if needed.

Take a moment to think about what your current mood level is on a scale of 1 to 10 where 1 is 'low mood', 5 is 'OK', and 10 is 'very happy'.

If your mood is 4 or below what are the warning signs? What are you going to do to lift your mood? What have you done before that worked? What will inoculate you in the future?

If your mood is 6 or above what did you do that made that happen? What is working well in your life? What can you learn from that? Can you do it again?

It is useful to keep a Positivity Journal to note all the things that work well for you. You can download a Positivity Journal template at www.hotwomencoolsolutions.com.

Confidence

Some women say that they felt like they became invisible once they turned 50; invisible at work, invisible in restaurants, and invisible to their partners. This can lead to feelings of frustration and unhappiness but there are many more positive examples of powerful older women—ask Madonna, Helen Mirren, or Goldie Hawn! It's often a case of your self-esteem.

A woman's experience at this stage of her life will be strongly influenced by her beliefs. We look for evidence to prove the things that we believe to be true. Beliefs come from many different sources, for example life experiences, parents, family, teachers, peers, society, books, and other media. They are powerful because we treat them as factual even though they rarely are.

Some beliefs are enabling, that is they can help you to achieve the results you desire. If your partner believes this is an exciting and liberating stage in her life she will have a positive experience. Other beliefs are limiting and they get in the way of the action you need to take. If you believe that your life will be all downhill after your fiftieth birthday, then you will notice all the things that reinforce that belief.

Enabling Belief	Limiting Belief
"I can control my menopause symptoms."	"There is nothing I can do. I just have to suffer."
"How I live my life will influence my experience of menopause."	"My menopause will be the same as my mother's—terrible!"
"I can ask if I need help."	"Asking for help is a sign of weakness."
"I can learn how to do whatever I want to."	"It's too late for me to learn anything new."
"We can try new things and enjoy ourselves."	"Our sex life is over now that we are getting older."

You can change limiting beliefs. One of the simplest ways is to act as if the belief isn't true. If you do that, you start to notice the evidence that it isn't true. Another technique is to identify the limiting beliefs and to create positive affirmations that will replace the negative messages that you are giving yourself.

Happiness at work.

Women who experience frequent or intense perimenopause symptoms may have problems in the work environment. These can have an impact on performance, attendance, and relationships at work.

If you think that your partner is experiencing problems at work, encourage her to discuss any specific issues with her manager even if that is a difficult or sensitive conversation. If she has a good relationship with her manager it should not be hard to broach the subject. If not, she will need to make arrangements for a discreet conversation at a time and place where they will not be interrupted.

It is important not to postpone this conversation until she is having an appraisal or performance review interview. She will need to stick to the facts about what she is experiencing and not to be too graphic. Encourage her to be clear about what action she needs her manager to take to assist her.

If the manager is uncooperative your partner may have to involve a trade union or welfare representative. There is legislation that can be applied to employees experiencing menopausal symptoms for example Health and Safety and Disability Discrimination acts.

Depending on the work your partner does and the nature of her workplace, the sort of issues she could discuss with her manager include:

- Workplace temperature and ventilation
- Proximity to windows
- Workstation design
- Standing duties
- Changes to uniforms

- Access to toilets and toilet breaks
- Adjustments to working time or duties.

Bullying and Harassment

Some women find that as they go through peri-menopause they become more sensitive to comments from colleagues at work referring to their symptoms. Men sometimes refer to 'women's problems' and make jokes about menopausal women because they feel embarrassed. However these types of comment and banter can be perceived as bullying and harassment.

This type of behaviour it can lead to loss of self-esteem, poor sleep, stress, anxiety, and depression. Therefore it is important to deal with it as quickly as possible either by discussing it directly with the person or people involved or by raising it with a manager. Do not let your partner suffer in silence.

CHAPTER 10

TEN TOP TIPS FOR A HEALTHY MENOPAUSE/ANDROPAUSE

If you have read the whole book you may have noticed some common themes. Here is a summary of the most important tips.

1   Be well informed. The better informed you are about what is going on in your body and your options for treatment, the better equipped you will be to obtain the resources you need.

a. Keep a record of the intensity and frequency of your symptoms.

b. Use this and other relevant books and websites to understand the risks and benefits of your treatment options,

2   Eat a healthy diet. Your experience of andropause, perimenopuase, and post-menopause will be significantly affected by what you eat—and don't eat.

     a. Eat lean protein, fruit, and vegetables.

     b. Limit your intake of carbohydrates, particularly refined carbohydrates such as white bread, white rice, and processed breakfast cereals.

     c. Avoid processed foods and 'fat-free' or 'low-fat' foods.

3   Drink plenty of water and non-caffeinated drinks. Staying well hydrated is important for your physical, mental, and emotional wellbeing. The diuretic effect of caffeinated drinks (tea, coffee, chocolate, and energy drinks) may flush vital nutrients out of your system. Substitute:

     a. Herb teas, fruit teas, or Rooibosch (South African caffeine free tea).

     b. Pure fruit juice diluted with mineral water.

n.b. Reduce your intake of caffeine slowly to limit the possibility of withdrawal effects.

4   Exercise. A mixture of resistance exercises and cardio vascular exercise will help to keep your body and mind healthy. Exercise is not confined to organised or gym exercises. There are opportunities to exercise every day at home and at work by walking a bit further, using the stairs instead of the elevator, or going to talk to someone rather than phoning or emailing. Remember, everything that you do more

than nothing could be the difference that makes the difference.

5 Adopt a healthy lifestyle—it's never too late to start. If you give up smoking today you will start to experience the benefits within a couple of hours. Within five years your risk of heart attack falls to about half of that of a smoker. Within ten years the risk of lung cancer falls to half of that of a smoker.

You do not need alcohol to have a good time. Reducing alcohol intake will reduce your calorie intake and help with weight control. It will also help you to control your moods and reduce hot flashes.

6 Keep your brain active. Getting older does not mean 'falling apart'! Staying involved and active as you age can slow down mental and physical degeneration. Keep challenging your brain by:
   a. Learning a new skill or language
   b. Changing your routine
   c. Getting involved in a volunteering activity
   d. Doing mental puzzles and quizzes
7 Consider food supplements. Even if you eat a well-balanced diet you may experience symptoms that could be alleviated through the use of food supplements such as multivitamins or omega-3 fish oils.
8 Sleep well. Your mind and body perform 'housekeeping' tasks during sleep that help to balance your hormones and keep your brain healthy. Everyone is different in how much sleep they need but you should aim for between 7–9 hours sleep a night.

Make sure that your bedroom is a 'sleep haven'—take out the television, computer, and mobile phone. Remember, if you wake up during the night don't reward yourself by getting up and doing anything interesting—rest, relax your body, and allow your mind to drift. If you must do something, have a drink of water and read something boring until sleep seems like a great option.

9 Control stress. The most important thing you can do to relieve stress is to take control of the situation. Even in the most difficult situations you always have options. Take time out to treat yourself even if it is only something small like having a five minute chat with a friend.

And finally:

10 Be positive. This can be the time of your life—but only you make it so. If you look for the negative things in your life you will find them and convince yourself that it's all bad. But if you look for the positive things you will find them and this will be a great time for you and those around you.

APPENDIX A: RESOURCES

Andropause Symptoms Record

If you think that you might be experiencing symptoms of testosterone deficiency, it is useful to keep a note of your symptoms that you can share with your medical practitioner.

Symptom	Yes/No	Frequency (per day or per week)	Intensity (scale of 1-5)
General fatigue			
Poor sleep			
Erectile dysfunction			
Loss of sexual appetite			
Weight change			
Low mood/ depression			
Hot flashes			
Night sweats			
Palpitations			

Menopause Symptoms Record

Your partner can use this table to keep a record of any menopausal symptoms that she is experiencing and anything that she has become aware of that triggers the symptom.

Symptom	Yes/No	Frequency (per day or per week)	Intensity (scale of 1-5)
Tension			
Mood swings			
Depression			
Forgetfulness			
Poor or interrupted sleep			
Weight change			
Headache			
Tiredness			
Dizziness or faintness			
Heart pounding			
Hot flash			
Night sweat			
Irregular periods			
Heavier/lighter periods			

Breast tenderness			
Abdominal bloating			

Links

You can access the following journals at www.hotwomencoolsolutions.com

- Menopausal Symptoms Journal
- Sleep Journal
- Food Journal
- Faulty Thinking Journal
- Positivity Journal

You can also download:

- Stay Cool Hypnotic/Relaxation Recording
- Mindful Weight Loss Hypnotic/Relaxation Recording
- E-book *Top Tips for Succeeding in Challenging Times*

Complementary and Alternative Therapies

For men and women who do not want to take prescribed medicines there is a range of complementary and alternative therapies that can help to relieve menopausal symptoms.

The best complementary therapies are holistic, that is they treat the whole person. They can generally be used alongside medical treatment but it is advisable to check with your medical practitioner if you are undergoing treatment.

When you are choosing a complementary therapist consider the following:

- Is the therapist qualified and insured?
- If you contact the therapist, do they welcome questions and answer them fully?
- Are they open about their fees?
- Do they have any testimonials on their website?

Be cautious about anyone who guarantees recovery or cures.

Aromatherapy

Aromatherapy involves the use of essential oils to provide a range of therapeutic healing benefits. Aromatherapy oils can be administered by inhalation or they can be combined with massage to provide benefits that range from stimulating to relaxing, depending on the individual's symptoms and goals.

There are a number of oils that can be used to provide relief from menopause symptoms including angelica, anise, basil, coriander, fennel, geranium, lavender, neroli, and sage. In particular, lavender is used for its calming effect which can be helpful for stress and emotional and mental symptoms.

Aromatherapy can be added to Vitamin E oil for massage treatments and this provides moisturising properties for the skin.
http://ifparoma.org/public/findatherapist.php

Nutritionists

Food supplements can be useful in supporting health though the perimenopause, even for women who are eating a healthy, balanced diet. Multivitamins combined with minerals specifically designed for menopause symptoms are available in pharmacies, health food stores, and on-line.

Omega-3 fatty acids are sold separately and are important for their anti-inflammatory action, helping with mood swings, and in reducing hot flashes.

For advice and supplements that are tailored to your symptoms you can consult a nutritionist.

UK http://www.findmynutritionist.co.uk/
USA http://www.findanutritionist.com/

Herbal Remedies

Herbal remedies can be helpful in alleviating menopause symptoms. Remedies can be purchased in pharmacies and food stores but for best effect it is advisable to consult a qualified herbalist.

Women taking herbal remedies should check the recommended period for taking them as many are only suitable for short term use.

Women who are taking other medication or who seek medical treatment should tell their doctor if they are taking herbal remedies.

UK: www.nimh.org.uk
US: www.americanherbalistsguild.com

Homeopathy

Homeopathic remedies can be helpful in easing meno–pause symptoms. A range of homeopathic products can be purchased in chemists and food stores but for best effect it is advisable to consult a qualified homeopathist. The appropriate remedy will depend on the individual patient and how they are experiencing the symptoms.

UK http://www.homeopathy-soh.org
USA http://homeopathyusa.org/

Hypnotherapy

Hypnotherapy has been shown to be effective in helping women who experience hot flashes, particularly when hypnosis includes visualisation of cool images. Women can be taught self-hypnosis so that they can take control of their symptoms. Hypnosis recordings are also very effective.

Cognitive hypnotherapy brings together hypnotherapy with Neuro Linguistic Programming (NLP) techniques, positive psychology and elements of cognitive behaviour therapy to provide treatment that can target particular menopausal symptoms including poor sleep, weight gain, and low mood.

UK http://www.cnhc.org.uk/pages/index.cfm
USA http://www.hypnotherapistregister.com
Cognitive Hypnotherapy www.questinstitute.co.uk

Reflexology

Reflexology is based on the principle that there are areas in the feet and hands that mirror each organ and structure in the body and they are connected to those organs by energy channels. Gentle but firm pressure is applied using thumbs and fingers on those areas. The therapist can induce a state of deep relaxation and trigger the body's self-healing ability.

Regular reflexology treatments can support a woman going through menopause physically, mentally and emotionally by identifying imbalances and treating areas which need attention.

UK http://www.cnhc.org.uk/pages/index.cfm
USA http://reflexology-usa.org/

Reiki

Reiki means "universal life energy" It is a Japanese healing treatment for balancing the energy system of the body. The practitioner places his/her hands in various patterns on the body using light therapeutic touch.

Reiki therapy can be used to treat common menopause symptoms such as hot flashes, insomnia, migraines, depression, and cramps.

http://www.iarp.org/

Shiatsu

Shiatsu is a massage therapy using the application of pressure on particular points of the body. Typically, pressure is applied while the client is lying down on a padded mat on a flat floor. The goal of shiatsu is to bring back the free flow of chi so that the body can come back into balance.

Prior to treatment, the practitioner will assess the client's symptoms, diet, lifestyle, and overall health. The effects of the treatment can be very calming and relaxing.

http://www.cnhc.org.uk/therapists/shiatsu-practitioners.htm

Traditional Chinese Medicine

Traditional Chinese medicine (TCM) originated in ancient China and has evolved over thousands of years. TCM practitioners use herbs, acupuncture, and other methods to treat a wide range of conditions.

In TCM the human body is regarded as an organic entity in which the various organs, tissues, and other parts have distinct functions but are also interdependent. In this view, health and disease relate to balance of the functions.

Acupuncture can be used to remove blockages or problems with the flow of energy around the body. Various approaches are used to stimulate points around the body including the use of fine metal needles to penetrate the skin. Although the idea of needles can be intimidating for some women, most find that the treatment is relaxing rather than painful. Typically, an acupuncturist will formulate a treatment plan after talking to the client about her specific menopause symptoms, diet, lifestyle, and overall health.

UK: Association of Traditional Chinese Medicine http://www.atcm.co.uk

US Accreditation Commission for Acupuncture and Oriental Medicine http://www.acaom.org

Acupuncture: www.acupuncture.org.uk and www.acupuncture.com

APPENDIX B: REFERENCES

www.nhlbi.nih.gov/whi/beckground.htm Women's Health Initiative

http://www.figo.org/news/losing-weight-may-reduce-symptoms-menopause-0010242 *Losing weight may reduce symptoms of menopause.*

http://blogs.plos.org/obesitypanacea/2011/06/22/does-weight-loss-influence-vitamin-d-levels/ *Does weight loss influence vitamin D levels? Travis Saunders, 2011*

http://www.sciencedaily.com/releases/2010/07/1007132 15202.htm

www.uq.edu.au/news/index.html?article=24445 '*Research allows doctors to predict menopause symptoms.*'

http://www.nejm.org/doi/full/10.1056/NEJMoa030311 2003, '*Effects of Estrogen plus Progestin on Health-Related Quality of Life*'

http://www.empowher.com/menopause/content/weight-loss-not-exercise-helps-night-sweats-and-hot-flashes-during-menopause?page=0,0 *Weight Loss, Not Exercise, Helps With Night Sweats and Hot Flashes During Menopause*

www.thelancet.com/series/physical-activity *Physical Activity* 2012

Achor, Shawn. *The Happiness Advantage,* 2010, The Random House Group

Chapman, Gary *The Five Love Langages; The Secret to Love that Lasts.* 1992 Northfield Publishing

Chiarelli, Dr Pauline, *Women's Waterworks – curing incontinence,* 1995 Khera Publications Ltd

Foxcroft, L., 2009 *Hot Flushes, Cold Science,* Granta Publications

Glenville, Dr Marilyn, *Natural Solutions to Menopause,* 2011, Rodale

Glenville, Dr Marilyn, *Fat Around the Middle,* 2006, Kyle Cathie Ltd

Gluck, Dr Marion and Edgson, Vicki, *It must Be My Hormones,* 2010, Penguin

Goodwin, J., 2012 *What Causes Hot Flashes, Anyway?* HealthDay News, April 12 2012

Gray, John, 1992, *Men are from Mars, Women are from Venus,* 1992, Harper Collins

Hamilton, Dr David R., *How Your Mind Can Heal Your Body,* 2009, Hay House

Harcombe, Z 2011 *Stop Counting Calories & Start Losing Weight,* Columbus Publishing Ltd

Hite, Sheer, *The Hite Report: A nationwide Study of Female Sexuality,* 1981, New York:Dell

Hollister, L. (1983), *'Treating depressed patients with medical problems'*

Lindenfield, Gael *'Assert Yourself'* 2001, Clays Ltd

Masters & Johnson, *Sex and Ageing – Expectations and Reality,* 1986

Ratey, Dr John J. and Hagerman, E. 2009 *Spark!* Quercus

Russell, J. 2005 *Can a vagina really buy a Mercedes? What can your pelvic floor do for you?*

Useful Books and Websites

<u>Andropause</u>

About.com, Senior Health
http://seniorhealth.about.com/library/usercontent/uc0408
01a.htm

Andropause Society, The Society for the Study of
Androgen Deficiency
http://www.andropausesociety.org/

AskMen (UK) for the Better Man
http://uk.askmen.com/sports/health_60/66_mens_health.
html

<u>Continence:</u>

ACA Association for Continence Advice
www.aca.uk.com

ACPWH Association of Chartered Physiotherapists in
Women's Health
www.womentsphysio.com

<u>Exercise:</u>

Couch to 5K - staged exercise programme for new
runners.
http://www.nhs.uk/Livewell/c25k/Pages/couch-to-
5k.aspx

Food Supplements:

Advice on food supplements and women's health issues:
http://www.naturalhealthpractice.com/

Hypertension:

American Society for Hypertension
http://www.ash-us.org/

British Hypertension Society
http://www.bhsoc.org/default.stm

Hypnotension TM – complementary approach to tackling high blood pressure:
http://www.hypnotension.com/

NHS UK
http://www.nhs.uk/conditions/Blood-pressure-(high)/Pages/Introduction.aspx

Hysterectomy:

www.hysterectomyconsequences.com

Listening skills

Tannen, D., *"You Just Don't Understand. Women and Men in Conversation"*, 1992, Virago

Tannen, D., *"That's Not What I Meant!: How conversational style makes or breaks relationships."*, 1992, Virago

Osteoporosis:

NHS UK
http://www.nhs.uk/Conditions/Osteoporosis/Pages/Introduction.aspx

National Osteoporosis Society in UK
http://www.nos.org.uk/

National Osteoporosis Foundation USA
http://www.nof.org/

Perimenopause:

UK
http://www.nhs.uk/Conditions/Menopause/Pages/Introduction.aspx

US
www.WebMD.com/menopause

US
www.fda.gov/womens/menopause

Relationships

Gray, Dr. J., *"Men Are from Mar, Women Are from Venus"*, 1992, HarperElement

Silvester, T., *"Lovebirds: How to Live with the One You Love"*. 2013, Coronet

General Menopause Websites:

For up to date advice and resources
www.shmirshky.com

The Change Explained
https://www.facebook.com/AlisonDotBrown

The North American Menopause Society
http://www.menopause.org/

Information about symptoms and treatment options
http://www.menopausematters.co.uk/

ABOUT THE AUTHOR

Pat Duckworth is a Cognitive Hypnotherapist, trainer, and author of the award-winning book, *Hot Women, Cool Solutions*. She has designed and delivered training in Neuro Linguistic Programming and a wide range of wellness subjects. She sees clients on a one-to-one basis in Harley Street and Hertfordshire and regularly runs training courses in Cambridge. She lives with her husband and cat in a small village in Cambridgeshire.

INDEX

Lightning Source UK Ltd.
Milton Keynes UK
UKOW06f2334110816

280536UK00019B/443/P